The Nervous System Reset

How to Harness the Vagus Nerve to Boost Energy, Focus, and Stress Resilience - The Science of Vagal Tone for Peak Performance in Work and Life

Nicci Brochard
&
Dr. Ben Chuba

The Nervous System Reset

How to Harness the Vagus Nerve to Boost Energy, Focus, and Stress Resilience - The Science of Vagal Tone for Peak Performance in Work and Life

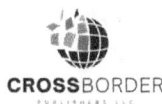

CROSSBORDER
PUBLISHERS LLC

New York, London, Quebec

Contents

Introduction

Your body possesses an extraordinary biological superhighway that directly connects your brain to every major organ—yet most people remain completely unaware of its existence. This neural pathway, known as the vagus nerve, represents the longest cranial nerve in your body and serves as the master controller of your autonomic nervous system. When functioning optimally, this remarkable nerve can transform your daily experience, delivering sustained energy, laser-sharp focus, and an unshakeable resilience to stress.

Modern neuroscience has revealed that vagal tone—the strength and efficiency of your vagus nerve—directly correlates with your ability to perform at peak levels. High vagal tone creates a physiological state where your body effortlessly shifts between activation and recovery, allowing you to tackle challenges with clarity while maintaining deep reserves of calm. Low vagal tone, conversely, traps you in chronic stress patterns that drain energy, cloud thinking, and leave you feeling perpetually overwhelmed.

The groundbreaking research emerging from leading universities demonstrates that vagal tone can be measured, strengthened, and optimized through specific, science-backed techniques. Unlike quick fixes or temporary solutions, these methods create lasting neuroplastic changes that compound over time. Elite performers across industries—

from Fortune 500 executives to Olympic athletes—have discovered that mastering their vagus nerve unlocks levels of performance they never thought possible.

This book distills cutting-edge neuroscience into practical protocols you can implement immediately. You'll discover evidence-based breathing techniques, targeted movement practices, and lifestyle adjustments that strengthen your vagal tone within days. More importantly, you'll learn to recognize and leverage your body's innate capacity for restoration and peak performance.

Your nervous system holds the key to unprecedented energy, focus, and resilience. The science is clear, the methods are proven, and your transformation begins now.

Nicci and I (Ben) thank you immensely for choosing our book. We promise you a wonderful time ahead.

Chapter 1

The High-Performer's Dilemma – Stress, Burnout, and the Brain

We introduce you to the age of burnout. The phenomenon of workplace burnout has become so widespread that the World Health Organization now officially classifies it as an occupational hazard, defining it by telltale symptoms of "exhaustion, cynicism, and reduced efficacy". In recent years, we've seen a dramatic wake-up call: what used to be worn as a badge of honor ("I only sleep 4 hours a night!") is now understood as a serious risk to both health and performance. In a 2021 survey of 1,500 U.S. workers, more than half said they felt burned out from their jobs, and an astonishing 4.3 million Americans quit their jobs in a single month at the end of that year, part of a "Great Resignation" fueled by burnout. The cultural tide is turning – even hard-charging CEOs have begun to admit that chronic overwork and stress are not the price of greatness but a "delusion" that ultimately backfires. Simply put, burning out is no longer a mark of toughness; it's a red flag that something needs to change.

Burnout is not "all in your head" – it literally leaves its mark on your body and brain. Mounting scientific evidence shows that the chronic, unrelenting stress behind burnout takes a profound physical toll, not just an emotional one. In fact, burnout is not just a state of mind at all, but a condition that can be measured in changes to our neurobiology. Researchers using advanced brain scans and hormonal tests have demonstrated that long-term workplace stress can overwhelm our body's normal stress-response systems and even lead to distinctive changes in brain anatomy and function. For example, people suffering from chronic burnout show alterations in key brain regions: studies have found that the frontal cortex – the area essential for memory, focus, and executive function – can thin prematurely in burnout patients, while the amygdala (the brain's center for fear and emotional reactivity) actually enlarges, reflecting a brain stuck in overdrive. In other words, extreme stress can physically reshape parts of the brain responsible for memory and decision-making. Far from being "all in your head," burnout lives in your nerve endings, your hormones, even the structure of your gray matter. No wonder it impacts so much more than just mood.

The Hidden Toll of Chronic Stress on Body and Brain

To understand how burnout wreaks such havoc, we need to look at the body's built-in stress response – an ancient mechanism honed by evolution. When you experience pressure or danger, your brain's alarm system (centered in the amygdala and hypothalamus) flips the switch on your sympathetic nervous system, triggering the famous "fight-or-flight" response. In the short term, this response is incredibly useful: it floods your bloodstream with stress hormones like adrenaline and cortisol, jolting you into a state of high alert. Your heart pumps faster, breathing quickens, blood rushes to your muscles, and your mind snaps into sharp focus. This acute stress reaction can be life-saving in the wild (springing you into action to escape a predator) and even beneficial at work – think of the burst of energy and concentration you might feel before a big presentation or deadline. A little acute stress can light a fire under you and boost performance.

The trouble brews when stress isn't a short-term burst but a never-ending state. In today's high-pressure world, many high-performers find themselves under *chronic* stress without adequate time to recover. The body's stress thermostat gets stuck in the "on" position. Over time, this continuous flood of stress hormones starts to wear down the system. The neuroendocrine system – particularly the HPA (hypothalamic–pituitary–adrenal) axis that regulates cortisol – can become dysregulated. At first, chronic stress might mean your cortisol stays constantly elevated; eventually, it may crash into abnormally low levels as your adrenal system gets fatigued from being overused (a bit like a car running out of gas). In either case (too high or too low cortisol for too long), the imbalance wreaks havoc on your health. It contributes to problems like persistent inflammation, lowered immunity, and even elevated risk of heart disease. If you've ever noticed that you get sick more often when you're burned out, this is likely why – your body's stress-response gear is malfunctioning, leaving you vulnerable.

Inside the brain, chronic stress sets off a cascade of changes that mirror this hormonal turmoil. Think of stress hormones like a fire alarm: in small doses, they wake the brain up; in large chronic doses, they start to damage the furniture. Elevated cortisol and other stress chemicals can interfere with the growth of new neurons and cause existing neurons to atrophy in crucial areas of the brain. Researchers have captured striking evidence of this "stress remodeling." For instance, brain imaging studies on professionals with severe burnout have shown shrinkage in parts of the prefrontal cortex (which we rely on for concentration, planning, and impulse control) and reduced connectivity in circuits that regulate emotion. One Swedish study of long-term occupational stress found that burned-out patients had a thinner medial prefrontal cortex (mPFC) – a region that normally helps keep us calm and focused – compared to healthy peers, as if their brains had aged faster under stress. The same patients showed an enlarged amygdala, suggesting their "fear center" was in overdrive, and even a shrunken caudate (a structure involved in learning and memory) correlating with their high stress levels. These anatomical changes paint a clear picture: burnout isn't just a vague feeling of exhaustion; it is physically etching itself into the brain's structure.

Beyond anatomy, scientists are finding that burnout leaves functional scars as well. Chronic stress seems to dull the brain's higher functions while amplifying primitive survival circuits. Have you ever felt so stressed that you *literally* can't think straight? That's not a figment of your imagination. Under unrelenting stress, the brain's executive center – the prefrontal cortex (PFC) – starts to lose its grip, while the reactive emotional centers (like the amygdala) run hot. Essentially, chronic stress can "hijack" the brain. This process has been observed in both humans and animals: psychologists note that tasks requiring complex, flexible thinking (a PFC specialty) reliably fall apart when someone is severely stressed, whereas simple, habitual tasks (more reliant on deeper brain structures) might hold steady or even improve. In one classic experiment, participants under an acute stress challenge (public speaking, a known stressor) showed impaired working memory and cognitive flexibility – both key PFC abilities – yet they paradoxically formed *stronger* fearful conditioning memories, which are linked to the amygdala. In short, high stress shuts down our brain's smart problem-solving region and lets the more primitive fear-driven region call the shots. Neuroscientists sometimes say that stress makes us rely on "habit over insight" – we become reactive and routine, rather than thoughtful and creative.

What does this brain hijack feel like in daily life? Imagine you're under intense pressure at work: deadlines looming, inbox overflowing. Initially, your sympathetic nervous system revs you up – you feel that adrenaline rush helping you focus. But as the stress drags on for weeks, you may notice you're losing sharpness. You start forgetting meetings, or you read the same email five times without absorbing it. That's your over-taxed PFC struggling to lay down new memories or pay attention. At the same time, you might find yourself on a hair trigger emotionally – little setbacks make you disproportionately angry or anxious. That's a sign your amygdala is now in the driver's seat. Indeed, research on occupational burnout finds it compromises our executive functions in everyday life. Burned-out professionals often report they "can't think straight," struggle with basic concentration, or make silly mistakes they'd never normally make. These aren't just subjective complaints: objective testing bears them out. In one review of studies, people suffering from burnout consistently performed worse on tasks of sustained attention, working memory, and cognitive flexibility compared to non-burned-out individuals. Even creativity and problem-solving – those higher-order thinking skills crucial for innovation — tend to deteriorate when burnout sets in. It's as if chronic stress narrows our mental bandwidth, leaving us with tunnel vision and a shorter fuse.

In line with this, many who have been through burnout describe a kind of mental fog. They might say, "I feel disorganized," or "I keep dropping the ball at work," or "I just don't have the mental clarity I used to." Clinical observations back this up: people with burnout frequently complain of memory lapses and trouble concentrating — for example, forgetting names, missing appointments, or needing to reread things — and studies show these issues can persist long-term if not addressed. Far from making us tougher or more productive, excessive stress undermines the very mental faculties that high-achievers pride themselves on. It's bitterly ironic: the harder you push yourself without rest, the more your brain pushes back by *shutting down* higher functions. Burnout is essentially the brain's way of forcing a hard reset when we've ignored all the gentler warnings.

Case Study: Arianna Huffington's Wake-Up Call

To put a human face on these concepts, let's look at a real-world high-performer who learned about burnout the hard way. Arianna Huffington — co-founder of the Huffington Post and now founder of Thrive Global — was for many years the very image of the always-on, success-at-all-costs executive. By 2007, Huffington was juggling the exploding growth of her media company and a hectic travel and speaking schedule, all while raising two daughters as a single mom. She later admitted she was working 18-hour days and getting by on as little as 3–4 hours of sleep a night, trying to "be superwoman" to everyone. To the outside world, she appeared to be handling it – the Huffington Post was a roaring success. But behind the scenes, her mind and body were wearing down from the chronic overload.

The breaking point came abruptly. One morning in April 2007, as Arianna was in her home office after yet another long night with almost no sleep, she collapsed. In a split second, she lost consciousness and fell face-first onto her desk, only waking up when she was already on the floor in a pool of blood. Disoriented and frightened, she realized she had blacked out from sheer exhaustion. The impact of the fall had broken her cheekbone and cut her eye – a serious injury. In the emergency room, doctors ran a battery of tests, thinking she might have had a heart episode or a neurological problem. But after ruling things out, the diagnosis that emerged was essentially extreme burnout: her collapse was the result of chronic sleep deprivation, stress, and overwork.

For Huffington, this was a defining wake-up call (quite literally). As she recovered, she was forced to reckon with the question: *What's the point of achieving great heights if you collapse in the process?* She later confessed that up until that collapse, she had bought into the same false belief that ensnares many high-performers – the idea that relentless hustle and self-neglect were the price of success. "I was working 18-hour days, trying to be superwoman, and it almost broke me," she said in hindsight. Lying in a hospital bed, she realized this approach was not sustainable. In her own words, "Something had to change – and it was me."

Huffington's rock-bottom moment led to a profound personal transformation. She began by making immediate changes to her lifestyle: she prioritized sleep and downtime for the first time in years, and instituted daily habits like meditation and unplugging from devices at night. As a Greek-born overachiever, Arianna also delved into wisdom from ancient philosophers and modern science alike, realizing that performance and well-being are not opposites, but deeply interconnected. Her journey culminated in her bestselling book *The Sleep Revolution*, in which she evangelizes the power of adequate sleep and rest as keys to productivity and creativity (not enemies of it). In 2016, she took the leap of stepping down from her role at HuffPost and founded Thrive Global, a company dedicated to ending the burnout culture and promoting science-backed strategies for wellness and peak performance. Through Thrive Global, and in countless speeches and articles since, Huffington has spread a clear message: burnout is not the price we must pay for success. In fact, she argues that avoiding burnout – through proper self-care, sleep, and recovery – is actually a prerequisite for sustained success.

Her story is a powerful reminder that even the most accomplished, ambitious individuals are not immune to the laws of biology. You can drive yourself only so hard, for so long, before the body says "enough." Arianna Huffington often notes that if you don't take time to recharge, your body will eventually force you to, whether through a collapse, an illness, or just a breakdown in performance. Yet her story is also an inspiring example that it's *possible* to bounce back and achieve even greater success by fundamentally resetting one's approach. After her recovery,

Huffington didn't fade away from the business world – on the contrary, she has arguably had an even wider impact by championing a new workplace culture that values well-being. The take-home lesson? Ignoring stress and burnout warnings can carry a heavy price, but heeding them can unlock even greater success. As we explore strategies in this book, remember Arianna's turnaround: it's never "too late" to course-correct and prioritize your nervous system's health. In doing so, you're not only taking care of yourself – you're also setting yourself up to perform at your peak for the long haul.

Stress vs. Performance – Finding the Balance

By now you might be thinking: "So should I eliminate stress entirely?" The answer is no – and, fortunately, you couldn't even if you tried. Some degree of stress is both inevitable and actually helpful in life. The secret that high-performers learn is not how to avoid stress altogether, but how to find the optimal balance of stress – enough to keep you motivated and engaged, but not so much that it overwhelms you. Think of stress like the tension on a violin string. With too little tension, the string produces a dull, off-key sound (or no music at all); with too much tension, the string can snap. But with just the right amount, that string can create a beautiful, resonant note. In the same way, zero stress can leave us unmotivated and underperforming – but excessive stress impairs our effectiveness and can "snap" our mental and physical health. Our goal is to help you tune your stress string to the right level, so you can play your best performance in work and life without fraying.

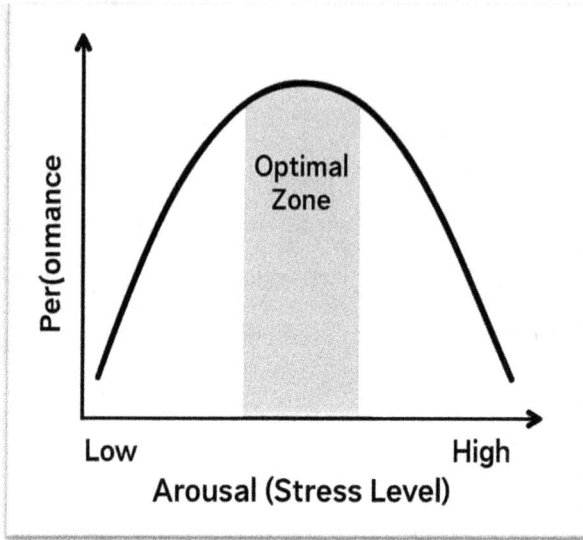

Figure above: The Yerkes-Dodson curve illustrates the classic relationship between arousal (stress level) and performance. Performance improves as stress/arousal rises from low to moderate (left side of the curve), reaching an optimal zone, and then declines if stress becomes too high (right side of curve).

In practical terms, a moderate challenge can energize and sharpen your focus — you feel "in the zone" — whereas chronic excessive pressure pushes you into diminishing returns, where you start making errors, feeling exhausted, or choking under the pressure. The key is to recognize when you're in that productive zone of stress versus when you're tipping into harmful overdrive.

Fortunately, your body and brain give off signals that can help you gauge where you are on that curve. Part of this guide will be about learning to read those signals — whether it's your heart rate variability, your sleep quality, your irritability level, or even your ability to laugh and experience joy. High-performers who sustain success learn to monitor these markers and adjust their approach before burnout hits. For example, slight stress might feel like butterflies in your stomach that motivate you to prepare for a big meeting – that's a healthy cue. But if you find yourself lying awake night after night with racing thoughts, or snapping at your loved ones because you're constantly on edge, those are warning signs that your stress has climbed too high.

The empowering news is that stress is manageable once you know how. The coming chapters will show you evidence-based strategies to keep yourself in balance – essentially, techniques to strengthen your parasympathetic "brakes" (the part of the nervous system that calms you down) so that after you rev up, you can reliably cool back down. We'll explore everything from the fundamentals – like sleep, nutrition, and exercise, which form the foundation of stress resilience – to advanced tools and "biohacks" for nervous system regulation. You'll learn how techniques like mindfulness meditation can literally rewire your brain for calm, how breathing exercises can tap into your vagus nerve to rapidly dial down stress, and how even things like cold showers or humming can stimulate your relaxation response. We'll dive into the science of vagal tone – a key measure of how balanced your nervous system is – and how improving it can boost your mood, focus, and energy levels. Importantly, we'll emphasize that resilience isn't about never experiencing stress; it's about recovering and resetting effectively. High performers use these tools not to live in a zen bubble, but to bounce back from challenges faster and stronger.

In summary, stress itself isn't the enemy. The real enemy is chronic, unrelieved stress – the kind that leads to burnout. The hero of our story is the often-overlooked counterbalance to stress: the power of deliberate rest, recovery, and nervous system regulation. By the end of this guide, you'll know how to harness the power of your vagus nerve and parasympathetic system to keep stress in check. You'll be equipped to maintain that optimal "violin string" tension, so you can perform at your peak without snapping. After all, sustainable success requires sustainable self-care – a truth that even the toughest high-achievers eventually come to recognize. In the chapters ahead, we'll show you exactly how to put that recognition into practice, using science-backed methods to reset your nervous system and unlock new levels of energy, focus, and resilience for both work and life.

So, as we conclude this opening chapter, take a moment to consider where you fall on the stress-performance curve right now. Are you feeling appropriately challenged and stimulated, or edging into overwhelmed and exhausted? If it's the latter, take heart. You're far from alone – and you now know that burnout is a real, physiological state that can be changed. The rest of this book is your roadmap out of the high-performer's dilemma. By understanding and applying the science of stress and the vagus nerve, you can break the cycle of burnout and find a healthier rhythm for sustained success. It's time to turn the page and learn how to reset your nervous system, boost your vagal tone, and thrive without burning out. Your peak performance journey is just beginning – and it starts with giving your brain and body the reset they deserve.

Chapter 2

Heart, Brain, and Performance – Listening to Your Body's Signals

You Can't Manage What You Don't Measure

High-functioning individuals live by the mantra, "you can't manage what you don't measure." In business, top executives rely on data dashboards to inform every decision. In much the same way, our bodies provide a constant stream of data – if we learn to listen. Consider your heart rate, breathing patterns, and other bodily signals as the analogs of a personal dashboard. By tracking these internal metrics, we can optimize our health and stress levels just as strategically as a CEO optimizes quarterly performance.

One powerful biofeedback metric gaining popularity among executives, athletes, and biohackers is Heart Rate Variability (HRV) – essentially, the variability in time between heartbeats. It might sound technical, but it's simply a measure of how consistently (or inconsistently) your heart beats over time. Why pay attention to HRV? Because it's a proxy for how balanced your autonomic nervous system is between "stress mode" and "recovery mode." In other words, HRV is like a check-engine light for your nervous system balance. Generally, a higher HRV indicates a calm, adaptable physiological state – your body's "engine" is running smoothly with plenty of flexibility – whereas a low

HRV can signal that your body is under stress or fatigue and stuck revving high in one gear. Research shows that having a high HRV reflects a robust ability to respond to changing demands, supported by strong parasympathetic (vagal) activity, which promotes mental clarity, focus, and stamina. By contrast, persistently low HRV often corresponds to an imbalance – typically too much "fight-or-flight" drive and not enough "rest-and-digest" – leaving the body less resilient.

It's important to note that low HRV isn't just about feeling stressed in the moment; it can also carry long-term health implications. Studies have linked chronically low HRV to increased risks of health issues like cardiac events, diabetes, stroke, and even higher mortality. In simple terms, if your HRV is consistently low, it's as if your body's stress brake (the vagus nerve) isn't working well, which over time can wear down your health. On the flip side, a high HRV is generally a sign of a well-tuned nervous system and better overall health – though "high" is relative to your personal baseline. While everyone's optimal HRV range differs, the key is that significant changes from your norm can tell you something. This is why elite performers treat HRV as an internal barometer, a way to listen to the body's signals and catch problems early.

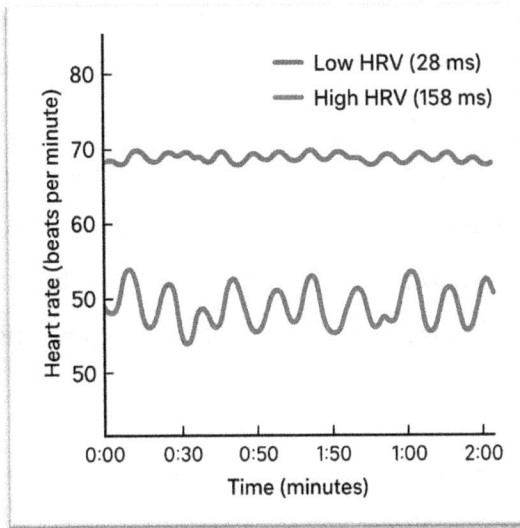

Figure above: Heart rate trajectories over two minutes for one individual on a day with low HRV (red) versus another day with high HRV (green). The red trace (low HRV of 28 ms) shows a higher, relatively steady heart rate around 70+ beats per minute, indicating a tense state. The green trace (high HRV of 158 ms) shows a lower average heart rate (~60 bpm) with more beat-to-beat variability, indicating a calm state with a responsive, flexible nervous system.

Notice how in the example above, the heart with high HRV is constantly speeding up and slowing down (a sign of healthy vagal tone), whereas the low-HRV heart beats more monotonously. At first glance, a steady heart rate might sound like a good thing, but in this context steady isn't better – it actually means the body has less adaptability. Think of HRV as the spacing between musical beats: a heart in a relaxed, adaptive mode plays a complex rhythm (variable intervals between beats), while a stressed heart marches on a uniform, relentless beat. The variability – the little fluctuations in timing – are a sign that the nervous system can smoothly toggle between states. In scientific terms, HRV is heavily influenced by the parasympathetic nervous system (particularly the vagus nerve). A strong vagus nerve input creates more variability between beats, so HRV is often considered a measure of vagal tone – essentially how effective your vagus nerve is at applying the "brakes" on your heart when needed. When vagal tone is high (high HRV), your body can downshift into recovery mode easily; when vagal tone is low (low HRV), your body has a harder time exiting the high-rev state of stress.

The Science of HRV: Tuning the "Gas" and "Brake" of Stress

What's happening under the hood to cause HRV to rise or fall? It all comes down to a delicate tug-of-war between the two branches of our autonomic nervous system (ANS). The sympathetic nervous system is the "fight-or-flight" accelerator – think of it as the gas pedal – and the parasympathetic nervous system is the "rest-and-digest" brake. These two branches are constantly sending opposing signals to your heart and other organs. Heart Rate Variability emerges from the interplay of these signals: when the parasympathetic (vagal) brake and sympathetic gas take turns effectively, your heart rhythm shows more variability. When one side (usually the sympathetic) dominates, the heart rhythm becomes more one-note.

To illustrate, consider what happens in a moment of stress. Say you're presenting at a high-stakes meeting or you hear sudden bad news – your sympathetic nervous system stomps on the gas. Your adrenal glands pump out adrenaline, your heart rate spikes, and your heartbeats become more uniform (fast and regular) as the body prioritizes pumping blood and oxygen to muscles. In this state, HRV plummets because each beat is coming rapidly and predictably on the heels of the last. Your body has essentially gone into high gear. In contrast, when you're safe and relaxed – imagine lounging on a porch on a calm evening – the parasympathetic system presses the brake. Your vagus nerve releases acetylcholine that slows the sinus node of the heart; your heart rate drops and, importantly, the timing between beats starts to vary more from one beat to the next. This high HRV state reflects a dynamic, resilient cardiovascular system that can bob and weave with life's demands. Neither state is "good" or "bad" in itself; you actually want a flexible nervous system that can hit the gas when needed and hit the brakes when the threat passes. Problems arise when we get stuck in high gear (sympathetic overdrive) for too long, or if our brake isn't strong enough to ever slow us down.

Scientists measure HRV in both frequency and time domains to parse out contributions of sympathetic vs. parasympathetic activity. Without getting too technical, high-frequency (HF) HRV components are mainly linked to parasympathetic (vagal) activity, while low-frequency (LF) components can include both sympathetic and parasympathetic influences (and are sometimes associated with blood pressure regulation and other factors). Under acute stress, studies show a very clear pattern: the vagal, high-frequency component of HRV drops off (since the brake is inhibited), and the relative power of low-frequency components often spikes, reflecting the sympathetic "fight-or-flight" surgepsychiatryinvestigation.org. A 2018 meta-review analyzed dozens of HRV studies and confirmed that in most people, induced stress causes a decrease in HRV, especially in those vagal-driven high-frequency fluctuationspsychiatryinvestigation.org. In other words, stress reliably puts the nervous system into a less variable, more locked-in state, which we can objectively see by measuring HRV.

Interestingly, our brain's stress circuits are tied into this process as well. Neuroimaging research has found that individuals with higher HRV at rest tend to have greater activation in brain regions like the ventromedial prefrontal cortex (vmPFC) – an area involved in emotional appraisal and regulation – when encountering stressorspsychiatryinvestigation.org. This suggests that HRV isn't just about the heart; it's a whole-body metric that mirrors what the brain is doing in stress processing. Essentially, a well-regulated brain (able to appraise and cope with stress) goes hand-in-hand with a flexible heart rhythm. Researchers have gone so far as to conclude that HRV is a useful objective indicator of psychological stress and overall health, given its consistent relationship with stress states and its ties to brain functionpsychiatryinvestigation.orgpsychiatryinvestigation.org. In clinical settings, doctors and psychologists are increasingly looking at HRV as a quantifiable window into someone's stress resilience.

To clarify the roles of the two ANS branches, consider the following breakdown of their effects on the body:

Sympathetic Nervous System ("Gas Pedal")	Parasympathetic Nervous System ("Brake")
Activates "fight-or-flight" response during stress.	Activates "rest-and-digest" response during relaxation.
Releases adrenaline and cortisol, increasing heart rate and blood pressure.	Releases acetylcholine via the vagus nerve, slowing heart rate and reducing blood pressure.
Dilates airways, increases blood flow to muscles, heightens alertness.	Stimulates digestion, promotes recovery processes (e.g. tissue repair, energy storage).
Reduces HRV (heart beats become rapid and more uniform under sustained sympathetic drive).	Increases HRV (heart beats slow down and vary more under strong parasympathetic tone).
Meant for short bursts of activity; chronic over-activation leads to burnout and fatigue.	Meant for long-term health; aids in calming the body and restoring balance (high vagal tone).

In a healthy, balanced autonomic nervous system, we seamlessly transition between these two modes. For example, during exercise or a challenging meeting, the sympathetic system takes the lead (HRV will drop in the moment); then during recovery or rest, the parasympathetic kicks back in (HRV rebounds). When we talk about improving vagal tone, we usually mean strengthening that parasympathetic brake – effectively training your system to relax faster and oscillate more easily back to a high-HRV state after stress. The remainder of this book will delve into exactly how we can do that. But first, let's see why people chasing peak performance are becoming obsessed with tracking this metric.

Why High Performers Track HRV

Imagine you're an Olympic athlete or the CEO of a fast-paced startup – peak performance isn't just about pushing hard, it's about balance and recovery. This is where HRV comes in. Many elite performers treat their HRV reading each morning like a personal status report on their recovery and stress levels. If you wake up and your HRV score is well below your baseline, that's essentially a red flag on your dashboard: something is off. Maybe you didn't sleep well, maybe you're fighting off an illness, or perhaps yesterday's workload (or workout) was more taxing than you realized. On the other hand, a high HRV score in the morning typically means your body is in a calm, primed state – all systems go for tackling challenges. In practical terms, HRV can inform decision-making: if HRV is low, high-performers might decide to take it easier that day, prioritize recovery activities, or employ extra stress-management techniques; if HRV is high, they might feel confident in pushing their training or tackling major tasks.

This approach to self-monitoring has become especially popular thanks to wearable devices that put lab-like measurements on your wrist or finger. Gadgets like the Oura Ring, WHOOP strap, Apple Watch, and

Garmin devices all offer HRV tracking. Every morning, you can receive a number (often part of a larger "readiness" or stress score) summarizing your heart's beat variability during the night. It's like waking up to a report card for your nervous system. In fact, a 2024 report in *Fortune* noted that "top CEOs are obsessed" with the Oura Ring and similar trackers, using them to gauge sleep quality and recovery status. Peek into boardrooms or the gym sessions of executives, and you'll notice these sleek rings and bands. The CEO of one social media giant and the co-founder of a major finance tech company have even been spotted wearing HRV-tracking rings, underscoring how mainstream this biofeedback has become among high achievers. The reason is simple: by paying attention to these internal metrics, they can catch burnout warning signs early and make adjustments before a breakdown occurs.

Let's consider a hypothetical case (a composite drawn from real stories of high-performers): An investment fund manager – let's call him Alex – starts wearing a WHOOP strap. On most mornings, Alex's HRV averages around, say, 80 milliseconds, which for him is normal. One month, during a particularly intense deal negotiation, he notices his morning HRV scores have plummeted into the 50s and 60s for a week straight. He also sees his resting heart rate creeping up about 5 beats above his usual. These are alarm bells. Even if Alex subjectively *feels* like he can force himself to power through (with enough coffee), the data is telling a different story: his nervous system is strained, stuck more in fight-or-flight. Taking the hint, he decides to postpone a non-urgent business trip that week and works from home for a day to rest up. He also schedules in a long nature walk and a few sessions of breathwork.

Sure enough, after a couple of lighter days and better sleep, his HRV readings climb back to baseline and his resting heart rate comes down. Alex likely dodged a bullet – by using HRV as an early warning system, he prevented a minor slump in readiness from snowballing into serious exhaustion or error on the job. This kind of self-regulation, aided by an HRV tracker, is increasingly common in the toolkits of executives and athletes.

There's also a competitive angle: What gets measured gets improved. High performers love to optimize, and watching HRV provides a concrete way to gamify recovery. If an executive notices that Friday happy hour drinks tank his HRV, he might choose to skip alcohol on days before important meetings. If an athlete finds that an extra hour of sleep boosts her HRV, she'll be motivated to hit the sack earlier before game day. In essence, tracking HRV helps connect the dots between lifestyle choices and physiological impact. It turns abstract concepts like "stress" and "recovery" into numbers you can watch, trend, and improve. No wonder it's caught on among those looking for an edge. As one performance coach quipped, wearing an HRV tracker is like having an executive assistant for your nervous system – it alerts you when you need a break, so you don't have to learn the hard way.

Burnout on the Radar: HRV and Chronic Stress

If short-term stress can nudge HRV down, what about long-term stress? This is where HRV's role as a canary in the coal mine really shines. Burnout – the state of chronic workplace stress and exhaustion – doesn't usually hit overnight. It builds up over weeks and months of imbalance.

By the time someone feels *truly* burned out (emotional exhaustion, persistent fatigue, cynicism), their body's systems have often been whispering warnings for a long time. HRV is one of those warning whispers that can turn into a shout.

Research has found clear differences in the HRV and heart rates of people experiencing clinical burnout versus healthy individuals. In one study of professionals, those diagnosed with clinical burnout had significantly lower waking HRV and higher resting heart rates than their healthy peers. In plain English, their bodies were stuck in high gear. The sympathetic "gas pedal" was floored and rarely letting up, resulting in a higher constant heart rate and very little of the healthy variability that comes from the parasympathetic brake. Imagine driving a car in first gear at 70 miles per hour – the engine would be screaming. That's akin to what these individuals' nervous systems were doing: running hot, with no efficient shifting or cooling down.

The same study also found that the burnt-out individuals showed differences in daily behavior, such as taking fewer steps per day on average than the non-burnt-out group. This makes sense: when you're chronically exhausted and stressed, you're less likely to be physically active (whether due to fatigue or lack of time for self-care). It becomes a vicious cycle – less exercise and movement can in turn further reduce HRV over time, since regular physical activity is known to improve autonomic balance. The researchers noted that burnout was linked with "alterations in cardiac physiology and physical activity in daily life," and suggested that these changes are easily detectable with wearable devices.

In fact, they concluded that continuous monitoring of metrics like HRV and daily steps could provide novel biomarkers of burnout, allowing for earlier intervention before someone hits the breaking point.

To put this into perspective, consider an anonymous case of a senior manager (we'll call her Maria) in a marketing firm. Maria prided herself on handling high workloads, but over a period of months she started feeling perpetually tired, and little health niggles were piling up. She began wearing an HRV-tracking ring after a colleague's recommendation. That ring became her mirror: it showed that not only was her HRV abnormally low most mornings, but her average heart rate during the day was 10 beats higher than it used to be. On top of that, the ring's app indicated she was only averaging 5,000 steps a day (on many busy days, much less), whereas healthy adults often aim for 8,000–10,000+. All signs pointed to a body under chronic strain. Armed with this data, Maria finally had an "aha" moment that her constant stress was quantifiably impacting her physiology. She took action – speaking with her supervisor about adjusting deadlines, incorporating short lunchtime walks (to get those steps up and clear her head), and practicing brief breathing exercises at her desk to stimulate her vagus nerve. Over the next several weeks, her HRV slowly improved and her resting heart rate edged down, tracking right alongside her improving mood and energy levels.

The good news is that wearable tech can catch these patterns and give you a chance to course-correct. If your device shows that your heart rate is consistently elevated and your HRV is chronically suppressed, it's a strong signal you might be in the burnout red zone. It's far better to heed these early warnings than to wait until you're so exhausted you have no choice but to take a prolonged sick leave. By listening to your body's signals – especially the ones as objective as HRV – you can take proactive steps to dial back stress before it becomes a full-blown crisis. In upcoming chapters, we'll explore specific techniques to boost your vagal tone and break the burnout cycle. But even before those interventions, the first step is awareness. This is where a simple practice of checking in with your body comes into play.

Practical Exercise: Check Your "Stress Pulse"

You don't need a PhD or a hospital lab to start tuning into your body's signals. Here's a practical exercise to build that awareness, using HRV or simple heart observations as a guide:

1. If you have an HRV-capable device: Begin observing how your HRV fluctuates day to day. Make a few notes for yourself correlating HRV with your circumstances. For instance, check your HRV on a high-stress workday versus a relaxed weekend. Note your HRV after a good night's sleep versus after a night of poor or short sleep. Many people discover clear patterns. For example, it's common to see that drinking alcohol in the evening will cause a noticeably lower HRV reading the next morning – a sign that your body is under internal stress while metabolizing the alcohol. If you have two glasses of wine at dinner, don't be surprised if your tracker flashes a warning the next day in the form of a suppressed HRV and elevated resting heart rate; this is your nervous system showing the impact of that extra load. On the flip side, try measuring after activities known to promote relaxation: perhaps do a 20-

minute meditation or take a gentle walk in nature one afternoon, and see if your HRV that evening or the next morning is higher than usual. Indeed, people often find that a mindfulness session or a peaceful hike can bump up their HRV, reflecting a shift into a more calm, parasympathetic state. The goal here isn't to achieve any particular number, but to learn the language of your own HRV – what makes it go up, what makes it go down – so you have a personal dashboard of what stresses or restores you.

2. If you don't have a fancy device: No worries – you can still listen to your body's signals in more basic ways. Try this simple check-in with your heart and breath, which we'll call the "stress pulse" exercise. Sit or lie down in a quiet place and place a hand on your chest or simply tune inwards. Notice your breathing rate and your heartbeat. Are your breaths coming fast and shallow, perhaps with a racing heart? That's a clue that you're in a sympathetic/stress state. Fast, shallow breathing often pairs with a lower HRV because you're effectively telling your body "we're busy or in danger." Now, take a minute to consciously slow your breathing – inhale deeply for a count of 4, exhale for a count of 6 or 8, letting the exhale be longer than the inhale. Do this for a few cycles and then observe your heart and breathing again. Most people will find their heart rate has decreased and each breath is deeper and slower – these are signs of the parasympathetic/relaxation response activating. You might even sense subtle variations in your heartbeat timing as you breathe (if you have a very keen sense, you can feel your heart rate slightly speed up when you inhale and slow down when you exhale – that's a normal phenomenon called respiratory sinus arrhythmia, a component of HRV).

By becoming attuned to these signals – your internal speedometer and breath rhythm – you are practicing the fundamental skill of body awareness.

Remember, awareness is step one in stress management. You have to notice stress signals before you can change them. This exercise of checking your "stress pulse" can be done anytime, anywhere: at your desk before a meeting, in the car (with eyes open, of course) during a traffic jam, or in bed at night. It's a way of taking your body's measurement in real time. Over time, you'll get better at catching yourself in a stress state early. For example, you might notice "Hmm, my heart is pounding and I didn't even realize I was that worked up about this email." That realization itself is powerful – it gives you a chance to intervene by maybe stepping away for a 5-minute break or doing a quick breathing exercise to reset.

In summary, listening to your body's signals – whether through technology like HRV monitors or through mindful observation of your heart and breath – is a game-changer for managing stress and boosting performance. By tracking a metric like HRV, high-performers gain an edge in self-care, making invisible stress visible and actionable. By practicing body awareness, anyone can learn to sense the early whispers of tension before they escalate into screams of burnout. In the next chapters, we will build on this awareness, exploring techniques to actively improve your vagal tone and enhance that heart-brain connection for peak performance. But none of those techniques will help if you're not first paying attention. So consider Chapter 2's lesson this: your body is always sending signals – start tuning in. Whether it's through a smart ring's data or the simple rise and fall of your breath, your heart and brain are in constant conversation, and you have the ability to listen and gently nudge the dialogue toward balance. By managing what you measure, you'll be on your way to a more energetic, focused, and resilient lifepsychiatryinvestigation.org.

Chapter 3

Sleep – The Ultimate Performance Enhancer

Sleep is arguably the ultimate performance enhancer for the human mind and body. In a culture obsessed with hacks and shortcuts, one fundamental truth stands out: nothing rivals the power of a good night's sleep for boosting your energy, sharpening focus, and fortifying resilience to stress. Not long ago, a hard-charging executive might proudly declare, "I get by on four hours of sleep," wearing it like a badge of honor. Today that attitude has flipped. Bragging about scrimping on sleep is now seen as a red flag – a sign of self-sabotage rather than strength. One prominent HR leader at a global company even remarked that claiming to thrive on 4–5 hours is essentially admitting you're harming your health and underperforming at work and home. In modern high-performance culture, chronic sleep deprivation isn't admired; it's viewed as a liability.

Why this change? Quite simply, sleep is not a luxury or lazy indulgence – it's a neurobiological necessity. If you want to operate at peak capacity, you must respect your nightly recharge cycle. Skimping on sleep is like running a high-performance sports car without oil changes – you might get away with it for a short burst, but eventually the engine will sputter. Leaders across industries have learned that sacrificing sleep in the name of productivity is a fool's bargain. The real power move is to *protect* your sleep, because it underpins every aspect of cognitive and emotional performance.

The Brain on Sleep: Overnight Upgrades

During high-quality sleep – especially in the stages of deep slow-wave sleep and rapid eye movement (REM) sleep – your brain is hard at work behind the scenes, performing critical upgrades and housekeeping. Think of deep sleep as the brain's maintenance window and REM as its creative studio. Here's what happens during those nightly cycles:

- **Memory consolidation:** Throughout the day you absorb new experiences and information, which are initially stored as short-term memories. During sleep, particularly slow-wave deep sleep, the brain replays and consolidates those memories, moving them into long-term storage. In essence, sleep is when your brain hits "save" on the day's learnings. Skip sleep, and it's like not hitting the save button – new information simply fails to stick. This is why pulling an all-nighter to cram for a presentation or exam often backfires: without sleep, much of that last-minute learning won't be retained.

- **Emotional processing:** REM sleep, the phase when vivid dreaming occurs, plays a key role in regulating emotions and stress. During REM, the brain's emotional centers (like the amygdala) and rational centers (prefrontal cortex) engage in a kind of overnight therapy session. Emotional memories get rebalanced and put into context, helping you wake up with a calmer perspective. Many people find that if they go to bed anxious or frustrated, the issue feels more manageable in the morning – you can thank REM sleep for that. When you shortchange your sleep, you rob your brain of this emotional reset, leaving you more reactive and less resilient to the next day's challenges.

- **Clearing out toxins:** Your brain has its own cleansing process called the glymphatic system. During deep sleep, brain cells shrink slightly, allowing cerebrospinal fluid to wash through brain tissue and clear out metabolic waste – including harmful proteins like beta-amyloid that build up during the day. In simple terms, sleep is when the brain takes out its trash. Consistently skimp on deep sleep, and those waste products don't get fully cleared, which may contribute to cognitive decline over time. This nightly cleaning is a big reason why after a solid sleep we feel mentally refreshed, whereas chronic sleep deprivation leaves the mind foggy and cluttered.

- **Hormonal reset:** Critical hormones follow a daily rhythm tied to sleep. During deep sleep, for instance, the body releases a surge of growth hormone – essential for cellular repair, muscle recovery, and metabolic regulation. Sleep also keeps appetite hormones in balance: going without enough rest boosts ghrelin (making you hungrier) and lowers leptin (making it harder to feel full), one reason people crave junk food when overtired. And then there's cortisol, the primary stress hormone, which normally dips at night and rises in the early morning to help you wake up. If your sleep is cut short or fragmented, this rhythm gets disrupted – you might find yourself wired late at night and sluggish in the morning. In short, a good night's sleep reboots your hormonal and metabolic systems, setting you up for stable energy and mood the next day.

All told, sleep is when your brain and body perform vital maintenance. If that nightly upkeep doesn't occur, things start to break down – fast. No wonder inadequate sleep wreaks havoc on nearly every measure of brain function.

The Cost of Cutting Sleep: Cognitive and Emotional Consequences

What happens when you don't get enough sleep? The truth is sobering: sleep deprivation hits the brain hard, undercutting your mental sharpness and resilience in ways you can't simply power through by willpower or caffeine.

Cognitively, short sleep is a wrecking ball. Attention and focus are usually the first to crumble – it becomes harder to concentrate, easier to get distracted, and you're more prone to errors. Your working memory (the brain's temporary "scratchpad" for information) grows unreliable, and your decision-making and problem-solving skills decline as well. In fact, staying awake for 20 hours straight can impair you as much as being legally drunk. For tasks that require precision – like performing surgery or driving a car – operating on insufficient sleep can be downright dangerous. And even if your job isn't life-or-death, sleep loss still causes sloppy work: think careless emails, missed details, poor judgment, and lackluster creativity.

Emotionally, a sleep-deprived brain is on a hair trigger. Lack of sleep amplifies the reactivity of the amygdala (your brain's fear and anger center) and weakens the logical control of the prefrontal cortex. In plain English, you're more likely to snap at colleagues or feel overwhelmed by minor frustrations when you haven't slept enough. Over time, this erodes your mental well-being. Chronic sleep deprivation is linked to higher rates of burnout, anxiety, and depression. It's hard to feel optimistic or resilient when you're running on empty.

Physically, poor sleep leaves you run-down. Your immune system is weaker (making you more susceptible to illness) and your appetite hormones misfire (making you crave comfort foods and making weight management harder). And of course, your energy levels plummet – everything feels more difficult when you're trudging through the day in a fog of fatigue.

Little surprise, then, that many workplaces now view chronic exhaustion as a liability rather than a virtue. These days, a bleary-eyed employee who burned the midnight oil isn't celebrated as a hero – they're seen as a potential risk to the team. Some companies even explicitly discourage the all-nighter culture, recognizing that well-rested employees simply perform better and more consistently.

How Much Sleep Do High Performers Need?

We've established that sleep is critical – but how much is enough? The optimal amount varies by individual, but large-scale research offers a useful benchmark. A study of thousands of adults found that about seven hours of sleep per night was the sweet spot for peak cognitive performance and good mental health. People who routinely got significantly less than that (say 5–6 hours or under) saw declines in attention, memory, and mood. Interestingly, those who regularly slept much more than 7 hours also tended to perform worse, suggesting there can be diminishing returns (or that consistently needing 10+ hours might signal poor sleep quality or an underlying issue).

For most healthy adults, experts recommend aiming for 7 to 8 hours of quality sleep nightly to function at your best. Some individuals feel great at 7, others need closer to 9 – there's room for personal variation. The key is to find the amount where you feel energetic, clear-headed, and resilient throughout the day. If you're dragging in the afternoon or relying on endless caffeine to get through, that's a sign you likely need more rest on a regular basis.

Notably, even ultra-busy leaders are coming around to protect this "magic" 7–8 hour window. One major tech CEO, for example, insists on about 8 hours of sleep every night. He believes any "productive" hours gained by skimping on sleep are an illusion, because the quality of his decisions would suffer. In his experience, important decisions and creative insights demand a well-rested brain, so he guards his sleep time accordingly. This perspective is increasingly shared by top performers across fields: at the end of the day, you can't cheat biology.

Sleep: The Secret Weapon of Elite Performers

Elite athletes and other high achievers treat sleep as a non-negotiable part of their regimen – a clear sign of its performance power. In professional sports, the conversation has shifted dramatically in the past decade. Teams and athletes now search for every edge, and prioritizing sleep has proven to be a game changer.

Take the case of one championship-winning basketball player who once struggled with inconsistency. Mid-career, he committed to better sleep – aiming for a consistent eight hours a night instead of the erratic, short sleep he used to get. The results were dramatic: his points-per-minute jumped by nearly 30%, his shooting accuracy surged, and his turnovers plummeted. When asked what made the difference, he summed it up: "Sleep more." That's coming from an elite competitor at the top of his game – proof that even when you're already excellent, better sleep can give you that extra edge that separates good from great.

Consider also the routine of a legendary quarterback with multiple championship rings. Despite being one of the hardest workers in sports, he famously enforces a strict lights-out bedtime around 8:30 p.m. Why? Because he knows that consistently getting his eight hours is key to his sustained success on the field, even as he ages. He credits prioritizing sleep as a secret to his longevity – while many of his peers burned out or faded, he was still racking up wins in his forties, thanks in part to the recovery and mental clarity that adequate sleep provided.

Olympians, too, are almost fanatical about sleep. One Olympic swimming champion, for example, tracks his sleep metrics as closely as his lap times. He and his coaches treat data on sleep quality and recovery as vital information guiding his training. If his tracker shows that his overnight recovery was poor, they adjust the next day's workout, knowing that pushing through fatigue could lead to injury or subpar results. Many Olympic teams now even hire sleep consultants and build nap time into training camps, understanding that when you're shooting for gold, you can't afford to neglect recovery.

And it's not just athletes. Across the professional world, top performers are discovering that sleep is their secret weapon. Some forward-thinking tech companies have installed nap pods for employees, acknowledging that a short midday snooze can do more for afternoon productivity than another cup of coffee. High-powered firms in consulting and finance are inviting sleep experts to coach their teams, trying to dismantle the old "all-nighter" culture. Even traditionally sleepless fields like medicine and the military have begun instituting stricter work-hour limits, because studies show that exhausted doctors and soldiers make more mistakes. In short, from the locker room to the boardroom, the smart money is on sleep.

Practical Strategies: Upgrading Your Sleep Routine

Understanding the importance of sleep is one thing; making sure you get high-quality sleep is another. The good news is that optimizing sleep is very much within your control, and small changes can yield big improvements. Think of it like crafting your personal sleep strategy – just as you'd strategize for an important project or athletic event. Here are some of the most effective, science-backed practices to upgrade your sleep routine:

- **Keep a Consistent Schedule:** Our bodies thrive on routine. Try to go to bed and wake up at the same times each day – yes, even on weekends. Keeping a regular schedule stabilizes your internal clock (circadian rhythm), making it easier to fall asleep at night and wake up feeling refreshed. If you constantly shift your sleep times – staying up late and sleeping in on weekends – you essentially give yourself "social jet lag." By Monday morning, your brain feels like it flew across time zones. Consistency is king: a steady sleep-wake pattern leads to better quality rest.

- **Morning Sunlight – Nature's Caffeine:** One of the simplest but most powerful habits for better sleep actually starts first thing in the morning. Get bright natural light soon after waking up. Exposure to sunlight in the morning (ideally within 30 minutes of waking, for about 5–10 minutes) sends a strong signal to your brain's clock. It triggers a healthy spike in cortisol (a hormone of alertness) to get you going, and it sets the timer for your evening melatonin release (helping you feel sleepy about 14–16 hours later). Even if it's cloudy, outdoor light is far more intense than indoor lighting – so step outside for a quick walk or have your coffee by a sunlit window. Think of morning sunlight as calibrating your body's internal clock; it's essentially free light therapy that can improve your sleep quality and daytime energy.

- **Create an Evening Wind-Down Ritual:** What you do before bed is just as important as your morning routine. In the last hour or so of your evening, start slowing things down. Avoid heavy mental work or stressful tasks – your mind needs a buffer between the business of the day and the onset of sleep. Crucially, minimize screen time during that final hour, especially blue-light devices like phones, tablets, and computers. Blue light tricks your brain into thinking it's daytime and can suppress the melatonin you need for sleep. Instead, dim the lights and do something calming. You might read a physical book, take a warm shower, do some gentle stretching or yoga, or practice relaxation techniques like deep breathing. The exact activity is up to you – what matters is that you have a consistent ritual that cues your brain it's time to unwind. Over time, your body will start to relax as soon as you begin your routine.

- **Optimize Your Sleep Environment:** Turn your bedroom into a sanctuary for sleep. Three big factors are darkness, quiet, and cool temperature. Make the room dark – consider blackout curtains or an eye mask, and cover any little electronic lights. Keep it quiet – if noise is an issue (loud neighbors, snoring partner, city traffic), use earplugs or a white noise machine (even a fan can help). And keep it cool – around 65°F (18°C) is often ideal, since your body's core temperature needs to drop to initiate deep sleep. Many people sleep poorly in a room that's too warm. Also invest in a comfortable mattress and pillow that suit your needs, since physical discomfort can sabotage sleep. The bottom line: you want your sleep environment to be soothing and free of distractions, so when you lie down, your body can fully drift into sleep mode.

- **Leverage Tech (but Wisely):** In our data-driven age, you might use a wearable or app to track your sleep. These tools can provide helpful insights. For example, you might discover that having a glass of wine or a heavy meal too close to bedtime significantly worsens your sleep quality and your recovery metrics the next morning. That kind of feedback can motivate you to change your habits (for instance, cutting off alcohol or big meals at least 3 hours before bed). However, a word of caution: don't become obsessed with chasing perfect sleep stats. There's even a term "orthosomnia" for people who get so anxious about hitting ideal numbers that they actually sleep worse. Use technology as a guide, not a gospel. Ultimately, how you feel in the morning is a better indicator of sleep success than any single number on an app.

By implementing even a few of these strategies, you'll be stacking the deck in favor of great sleep. And when you prioritize sleep, it's like compounding interest for your body and brain – each good night builds on the last, steadily boosting your daytime performance.

The Payoff: Resilience, Clarity, and Peak Performance

It bears repeating: sleep is the rising tide that lifts all boats in terms of mental and physical performance. It's been called the Swiss Army knife of health for good reason. Get enough sleep and you improve in almost every way: your memory sharpens, your creativity blooms, your mood steadies, your immune system strengthens – and your stress resilience skyrockets. This last point is key: when you're well-rested, you're far less reactive to stress. Small problems stay small; you can respond thoughtfully rather than overreacting. Physiologically, quality sleep tunes up your parasympathetic nervous system (largely driven by the vagus nerve), which is your body's calming, restorative mode. Good sleep often shows up as a higher heart rate variability and a lower resting heart rate – signs that your nervous system is balanced and resilient. In other words, sleep is a nightly reset for your brain and body, leaving you better equipped to handle whatever challenges come your way.

In the pursuit of peak performance – be it in the boardroom, in a creative project, or any high-pressure arena – it's easy to think you should grind longer and sleep less to get ahead. But the science and the habits of high performers say otherwise: often the smartest move you can make is to protect your sleep time. As the saying goes, "Sleep is the greatest legal performance-enhancing drug." And unlike a drug, it's free and good for you!

So the next time you're tempted to stay up late to "get more done," remember that you'll get far more done – with better quality – after a proper night's rest. Sleep truly is the foundation upon which all other strategies for health and performance stand.

Embrace it. Treat your sleep with the respect an elite athlete or world-class CEO would – as sacred recovery time. By doing so, you'll make smarter decisions and show up as the best version of yourself in work and life.

Tonight, give yourself permission to shut down the laptop, dim the lights, and turn in a bit earlier. You're not wasting time – you're investing in your performance. The path to unlocking your highest potential just might begin with a good night's rest.

Chapter 4

Train Your Brain – Mindfulness and Stress Resilience

Imagine if there were a pill that could increase your focus, improve your emotional self-control, and lower your stress – with virtually no side effects. It doesn't exist in pharmacies, but there *is* a practice that matches this description: mindfulness meditation. Once dismissed as a "new-age" fad, mindfulness has gone fully mainstream, especially among high-performers. We've reached a point where CEO after CEO openly credits their meditation practice as a key to their effectiveness and sanity. In fact, many top leaders and entrepreneurs – from Arianna Huffington and Oprah Winfrey to LinkedIn's Jeff Weiner and Bridgewater's Ray Dalio – are all reported to meditate regularly. Entire companies have embraced mindfulness programs as well, from Google and Nike to Goldman Sachs. When so many busy, results-driven people make time to sit quietly with their eyes closed, you know something important is happening. Mindfulness is no longer just a wellness buzzword; it's becoming a secret weapon for peak performance.

What Is Mindfulness Meditation?

So, what exactly *is* mindfulness? In essence, mindfulness is mental training to focus on the present moment, usually by anchoring attention (for example, on the breath or bodily sensations) and calmly observing thoughts or feelings without getting carried away by them. Think of it as doing focused "reps" for your attention span. Just like lifting weights strengthens a muscle, repeatedly bringing your wandering mind back to a point of focus strengthens neural circuits in the brain associated with attention and emotional regulation. Over time, this practice trains you to become both more concentrated and more emotionally steady.

At its core, mindfulness is about paying attention to what's happening *right now* – on purpose and without judgment. You might focus on the cool air entering your nostrils and the warm air flowing out, or the sensation of your feet on the floor. Inevitably, your mind will start wandering (did you reply to that email? what's for dinner? oh, that meeting tomorrow...). When it does, instead of scolding yourself, you simply notice the thought and gently return your attention to the present (the breath, the feet, the sounds around you, etc.). This simple cycle of distraction and return, done over and over, is the mental workout. Each "rep" is like a bicep curl for your brain's attention centers. Over time, it can literally grow your "mental muscle."

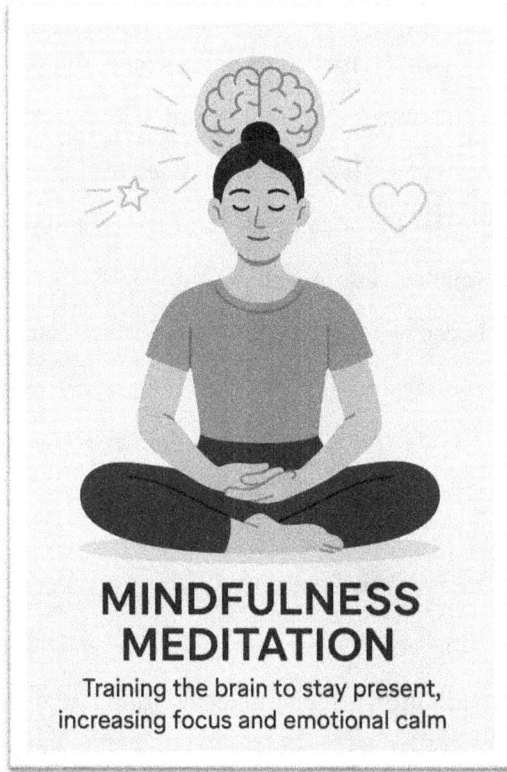

MINDFULNESS MEDITATION
Training the brain to stay present, increasing focus and emotional calm

This isn't just spiritual talk; a wealth of scientific research backs up the cognitive benefits. Even brief mindfulness training in novices has been shown to boost focus and cognitive performance. For example, in one study, people who did a mere 10-minute guided meditation performed better on attention tasks immediately afterward compared to a control group. In another experiment, just eight weeks of short daily meditations led to improved working memory and recognition memory in participants. These findings suggest that you don't need years of practice to see benefits – *even a few minutes of mindfulness can tune up your brain's focusing ability.* Long-term meditators, those with years of practice, often show even more dramatic enhancements. Seasoned meditators tend to exhibit superior memory and stress management capacity compared to non-meditators. In fact, brain scans reveal that long-term meditation is associated with physical changes in the brain: for instance, meditators have a larger hippocampus, the region crucial for memory and learning, and a smaller, less reactive amygdala, the brain's fear and emotion center. These structural changes correlate with better memory retention and a calmer baseline mood. It appears that by practicing mindfulness, people are literally reshaping their brains for better focus and resilience.

The Science: How Meditation Changes Your Brain

What's happening under the hood? Modern neuroscience has begun to map out how meditation affects brain function and wiring. It turns out meditation works, in part, by increasing activity in key "executive" areas of the brain – like the prefrontal cortex (PFC) and anterior cingulate cortex (ACC) – while dialing down reactivity in the amygdala. The PFC and ACC are responsible for attention, decision-making, and self-control, and studies show these regions become more active and even grow in gray matter density with regular meditation. At the same time, the amygdala (the alarm bell for stress and fear) tends to become less reactive and even physically smaller in meditators. One review noted that mindfulness practice can lead to reduced size and reactivity of the amygdala, aligning with reports that meditators have a more subdued stress response. In practical terms, this means that meditation is strengthening the neural circuitry for focus and calm, while quieting the circuitry for fear and stress. It's like increasing the signal of a wise inner coach in your mind (the PFC) and lowering the volume on the panicky inner critic (the amygdala). No wonder meditators often report feeling more *centered* and less easily thrown off by challenges.

These brain changes translate into real-world performance boosts. Research has documented improvements in executive functions – skills like attention control, decision-making, and cognitive flexibility – among those who meditate. Even novices show gains: a 2018 study found that after a single 10-minute mindfulness session, participants had better accuracy and quicker response times on cognitive tasks than those who didn't meditate. Long-term practitioners frequently demonstrate enhanced abilities to sustain attention and switch between tasks efficiently. There's also evidence for improved creativity and problem-solving, likely because a calmer, more focused mind can enter "flow" states more readily and think outside the box. Many high achievers say some of their best ideas surface during or after meditation – indeed, Ray Dalio has noted that his twice-daily meditation often leaves him with creative insights and clarity he didn't have before.

Crucially, meditation isn't about escaping or tuning out the world. It's about training your mind so you can engage with life more effectively. By practicing staying present and non-reactive during meditation, you're better equipped to do the same when life throws a curveball. This becomes most apparent in how mindfulness affects our response to stress – a topic especially relevant to avoiding burnout and sustaining peak performance.

Stress Reduction and Emotional Resilience

Perhaps the most celebrated benefit of mindfulness is its power to help you respond to stress more skillfully. Life will always have stressors – tight deadlines, unexpected crises, difficult conversations – but how you *handle* them can make all the difference. Mindfulness teaches you to cultivate a mental "buffer," a slight pause between a stimulus and your response. Instead of immediately reacting in a knee-jerk way (panicking, yelling, or shutting down), a mindful brain learns to take a beat. In that brief space, you can assess the situation and choose a more thoughtful response. As the famous psychiatrist Viktor Frankl said, *between stimulus and response there is a space, and in that space lies our freedom.* Mindfulness helps you find that space.

Over time, this non-reactivity becomes a habit. Say an urgent work email arrives: rather than your heart rate spiking and stress spiraling as you *instantly* start catastrophizing, you might notice the initial jolt of anxiety ("Okay, I feel my chest tighten, my mind racing") and then take a slow breath. That moment of awareness can prevent the snowball of stress from rolling downhill. You gain a sort of emotional equilibrium – an ability to stay grounded under pressure. This is not just anecdotal: studies show meditators have significantly lower emotional reactivity. Their amygdala (the fight-or-flight trigger) fires less intensely, and their prefrontal cortex steps in to keep them composed. In practical terms, mindfulness practitioners are less likely to "fly off the handle" when provoked and more likely to keep their cool and think clearly.

The physiological effects are significant too. Regular meditation is correlated with *measurably* lower stress hormones and a calmer nervous system. For instance, people who complete mindfulness programs often have lower baseline cortisol levels, the hormone associated with chronic stress. One long-term study found that participants who increased their mindfulness through meditation had decreases in their resting cortisol over time – indicating a more relaxed physiological state. Meditation also appears to shift the balance of your autonomic nervous system toward the parasympathetic side – the "rest and digest" mode. In other words, it activates your vagus nerve and increases your vagal tone, putting you into a calmer state more often. This shows up in metrics like heart rate variability (HRV), which tend to improve with deep breathing and meditation. Higher HRV (a sign of strong vagus nerve activity) means your body can flexibly dial down stress responses and recover quickly. In plain language, meditation strengthens your relaxation response – a term Harvard researcher Dr. Herbert Benson coined decades ago – which is the polar opposite of the fight-or-flight response.

And the benefits extend to the workplace in a big way. When employees practice mindfulness, they become more resilient against burnout. In fact, one comprehensive meta-analysis of 56 studies found that mindfulness-based programs in the workplace significantly reduce stress and burnout among employees, while improving their overall well-being and even job satisfaction. The effect sizes ranged from small to large, but the consistent finding was clear: calmer, more mindful employees are less exhausted and more content. They even showed fewer physical stress symptoms and somatic complaints. Another review noted that mindfulness training at work led to improvements in compassion and emotional health of employees – which isn't just "soft stuff," but translates to better teamwork and leadership. In short, a mindful workforce can handle challenges without hitting the panic button as often, and that equates to a more sustainable, productive work environment.

Case Study: Aetna's Mindfulness Revolution

One of the most dramatic real-world examples of mindfulness in action comes from insurance giant Aetna under the leadership of CEO Mark Bertolini. Bertolini's journey is fascinating: after a near-fatal skiing accident left him with a broken neck and chronic pain, he found that *conventional* medicine (and a cocktail of narcotic painkillers) wasn't helping him enough. Desperate for relief, he ventured into alternative therapies like yoga and meditation – and it worked. The practices significantly reduced his pain and improved his outlook. By 2010, when he became Aetna's CEO, Bertolini was convinced that these mind-body techniques could benefit everyone, not just patients or yogis. He decided to bring mindfulness into the corporate culture.

Bertolini introduced free mindfulness and yoga classes for Aetna employees, even allowing them to take these classes on the clock. Skeptics wondered if employees would sign up or if this was just a feel-good gimmick. The results blew everyone away. More than 13,000 Aetna employees (out of ~50,000) voluntarily participated in the mindfulness training – a huge uptake. And those who did reported striking improvements in their well-being. On average, these employees had a

28% reduction in their stress levels, a 20% improvement in sleep quality, and a 19% decrease in their perception of pain. These aren't small tweaks; they're life-changing differences. Think about that – over a quarter less stress!

The benefits didn't stop at personal health. Aetna noticed that employees who took the mindfulness classes became *more effective* at work. How do you measure that? One way is time – participants gained about 62 minutes of extra productive time per week, on average. Instead of losing an hour to stress, distractions, or fatigue, they *gained* an hour of clear-headed productivity. Aetna's analysts calculated that this was worth about $3,000 per employee per year in output. When multiplied across thousands of employees, that's a serious ROI for just teaching people to breathe and focus. Even Aetna's healthcare costs saw an impact: the year after rolling out the mindfulness program, the company's healthcare expenses actually fell by 7% (saving about $9 million), bucking the trend of rising costs. While Bertolini was careful to note that multiple wellness initiatives contributed to this drop (they also had weight-loss and exercise programs), he believes meditation and yoga played a significant role.

This case is inspiring because it shows the tangible, dollars-and-cents benefits of mindfulness on a large scale. We often talk about stress reduction in abstract terms, but here it increased profits, saved money, and created happier employees. And importantly, it started from the *top*: a CEO who had experienced the power of mindfulness firsthand became a champion for bringing humanity into the workplace. As Bertolini put it, "We have this groundswell inside the company of people wanting to take the classes... It's been pretty magical,". Magical indeed – but it's also just physiology and psychology working together. Lower stress and better sleep make people more energetic and engaged. Focused minds make fewer mistakes. Calm leaders make better decisions. The Aetna story is a blueprint for how mental well-being and corporate success can go hand in hand.

Not all of us have on-site meditation classes or a CEO who's a yogi, but the lesson here is that even in a high-pressure corporate setting, mindfulness can dramatically improve performance metrics *and* quality of life. Whether you're a manager or an individual contributor, this is food for thought: perhaps training the brain is a smart investment, not a luxury. Next, let's look at how *you* can start training your brain in mindfulness, no matter how busy your schedule might be.

Practicing Mindfulness: Quick Exercises to Train Your Brain

You don't need to sit on a cushion for hours or transform into a monk to reap the benefits of mindfulness. In fact, micro-practices woven into your day can be incredibly effective. Below are a few accessible exercises to get you started. These techniques act like *mental workouts* or reset buttons you can press whenever stress builds up or you find your focus flagging. Think of them as tools for your performance toolkit – use them at work, at home, whenever you need a mental boost or a moment of calm.

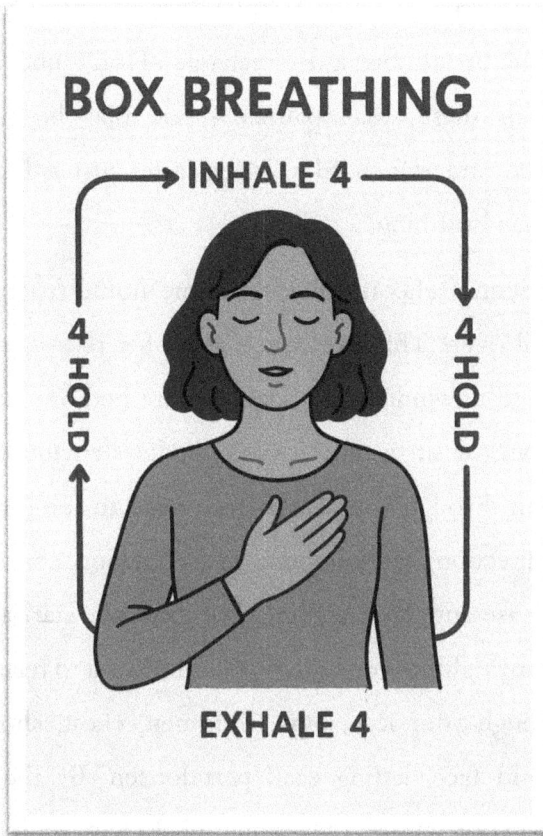

Figure above: Mindful breathing techniques, like "box breathing," quickly calm the body's stress response and clear the mind for better focus.

- **The 5-Minute Breath Break:** Start (or break up) your day with just five minutes of focused breathing. Sit comfortably, close your eyes, and pay attention to your breath – notice the cool air flowing in, the warm air flowing out. If your mind wanders (and it *will*), gently guide your attention back to the breath without any frustration. This simple exercise, done consistently, builds mental focus over time. It's like hitting a mental "reset" button.

Whenever you feel overwhelmed during the day, you can take a 5-minute breath break to recharge. Don't underestimate the power of these small pauses – you may be surprised how refreshed and refocused you feel after just a few minutes of conscious breathing.

- **Body Scan Relaxation:** Ever come home from work feeling tense all over? This exercise is great for releasing accumulated stress and unwinding, especially before bed or after a long day. Lie down (or sit back in a chair) and systematically move your attention through your body from head to toe (or toe to head, either direction). As you focus on each region, consciously soften and release any tension there. For example, start at your toes – notice any tightness or sensation, and allow it to relax. Then move up through your legs, hips, abdomen, chest, shoulders, arms, neck, and face, letting each part loosen. By the time you've scanned your whole body, you'll likely feel significantly calmer and more "in your body" rather than stuck in your whirling thoughts. Many guided body scan meditations (10–20 minutes long) are available on apps like Headspace or Calm, which can be helpful if you prefer a voice to lead you. This practice not only relaxes you, it also hones your ability to pay attention to subtle sensations – a key aspect of mindfulness.

- **Mindful Moments in Daily Life:** Mindfulness doesn't only happen in formal meditation. You can weave awareness into ordinary activities and turn them into mini-meditations. For instance, when you drink your morning coffee or tea, *just drink it.*

Don't multitask or scroll through your phone at the same time. Instead, take that short time to really experience the drink – feel the warmth of the mug in your hand, inhale the rich aroma, savor the taste of each sip. Be fully present with that simple act. Or try this: every hour or two at work, take a 60-second mindfulness pause. Push back from your desk, close your eyes (or soften your gaze), and do a quick check-in: notice any tightness in your body (maybe your shoulders or jaw), notice your mood, and take a few deep breaths. You could also stand up and stretch slowly, observing how it feels. These tiny moments of mindfulness sprinkled through the day act like pressure release valves, preventing stress from snowballing. They also refocus your mind, so you're sharper for the next task. Over time, you'll find that these little practices cultivate a steadier, more attentive mind all day long.

- **Box Breathing for Immediate Calm:** When the pressure is on and you feel anxiety rising – heart racing, mind chattering – box breathing is a clutch technique to regain calm quickly. This method is so effective that it's a favorite of the U.S. Navy SEALs for staying cool under extreme stress. *Box breathing* involves a four-part breath, each part of equal length (like the four sides of a square): inhale for a count of 4, hold your lungs full for 4, exhale for 4, hold your lungs empty for 4, then repeat. Just a few minutes of this can do wonders for your physiology. Research shows that controlled breathing techniques like this can rapidly lower heart rate and blood pressure by activating the vagus nerve and calming the autonomic nervous system. Essentially, by holding and slowing your breaths, you increase carbon dioxide slightly in your blood, which triggers a reflex that *slows* your heart and stimulates the relaxation response. The result? Within a couple of minutes, you shift from the adrenaline-fueled fight-or-flight state into a calmer mode. Box breathing also sharpens your mental focus, clearing away jittery energy and aligning your mind on a single task (counting and breathing). In fact, many people report that after doing 5–10 rounds of box breathing, they feel not only calmer but also more alert and concentrated than before. The beauty of this technique is that it's incredibly portable – you can do it quietly at your desk before a big meeting, in your car before an interview, or even in the bathroom if you need a private moment to compose yourself. The next time you notice panic or anger beginning to spike, try "boxing" your breaths. You'll likely be amazed at how effectively this can interrupt the stress response and reset your mood. *(Pro tip: if a count of 4 feels too easy after a while, you can extend to counts of 5 or 6 for a deeper challenge. And remember, breathing through your nose (on inhales) can help engage the diaphragm more fully.)*

World Inspiration: Ray Dalio's Meditation Habit

To really drive home how powerful training your mind can be, let's revisit one of the high-performers mentioned earlier: Ray Dalio. Dalio is the billionaire investor who founded Bridgewater Associates, one of the world's largest and most successful hedge funds. He's known on Wall

Street for his sharp analytical mind and unflappable demeanor in chaotic markets. What's his secret? According to Dalio himself, it's not an Ivy League degree or a superhuman work ethic – it's meditation. *"Meditation, more than anything in my life, was the biggest ingredient of whatever success I've had,"* Dalio said. That's a stunning statement if you think about it: a man who manages billions of dollars, crediting daily meditation as the top factor in his achievements.

Dalio has been practicing Transcendental Meditation (TM) since 1968, long before mindfulness was trendy. He maintains a strict routine: two sessions of 20 minutes each day, like clockwork – often once in the morning and once in the afternoon. He treats these sessions as non-negotiable appointments with himself. In interviews, he's mentioned that each meditation feels like a "20-minute vacation" that leaves him calmer and clearer-headed. Think about that: twice a day, he effectively gives himself a refreshing mental vacation, no exotic beach required. Dalio finds that after meditating, he's more creative and makes better decisions. In the high-stakes world of hedge funds, a single insight or a moment of clarity can be worth millions – so it's fascinating that he deliberately carves out time to sit in silence, because he knows it pays dividends in mental performance.

And he's not alone. Many other leaders echo the sentiment that training the mind gives them a real edge. For example, Salesforce founder Marc Benioff has been vocal about his meditation practice, even building dedicated meditation rooms at Salesforce offices for employees. Media mogul Oprah Winfrey has long championed meditation and often starts her day with it, even encouraging her staff at OWN network to meditate together. The late Steve Jobs was deeply into Zen mindfulness and credited it with helping him think clearly and design with focus. Athletes, too, have jumped on board: NBA coach Phil Jackson taught mindfulness to his championship-winning Chicago Bulls and LA Lakers teams, and players like Kobe Bryant and LeBron James have practiced meditation to enhance their game. From the trading floor to the basketball court, those who train their brain with mindfulness seem to gain a secret advantage – better concentration, better emotional resilience, and a calmer mind under stress, which all translate to superior performance in their field. As Dalio famously advised, if he could give one piece of advice to anyone, it would be to meditate, because of the calm and equanimity it provides.

This isn't to put these folks on a pedestal, but rather to show that mindfulness is a tool for everyone, not just mystics or monks. High-powered executives, creatives, athletes, and everyday people are all using it to navigate life's challenges more effectively. You might not have 40 minutes a day for meditation like Ray Dalio (and that's okay!), but even a fraction of that time can start shifting things for you. The key is to make it a regular habit – consistency is more important than duration. Whether it's five minutes in the morning, a short breather at lunch, or a routine of mindful prayer or reflection at night, *training your mind* is absolutely worth the time investment.

The Takeaway: Mental Fitness for Peak Performance

The big takeaway from all of this is that mental fitness is just as crucial as physical fitness for sustained high performance. We live in a world where we routinely schedule workouts for our bodies – we lift weights, go for runs, do yoga – recognizing that these practices keep us strong and healthy. It's time we give our brains and nervous systems the same level of care. Mindfulness, meditation, deep breathing exercises, prayer, or any form of intentional mental training can be thought of as "gym sessions" for your brain. They build up your concentration "muscles," flex your stress-response "resilience," and polish your emotional balance. In the same way cross-training your body with cardio and strength makes you an all-around better athlete, cross-training your mind with focus practices, relaxation techniques, and self-awareness makes you an all-around more effective human being.

And these practices are not just "nice-to-have" stress reducers; they are productivity tools, creativity boosters, and in the long run, burnout preventers. By improving your vagal tone and keeping your nervous system more often in a state of balance, you prevent the wear-and-tear that chronic stress inflicts on your body and mind. That means more energy available for what matters to you, whether it's strategic thinking at work or being present with your family at home. When challenges arise – and they always will – a trained mind handles them with more grace and less turmoil. You can work hard and pursue ambitious goals without running yourself into the ground, because you have the self-regulation tools to recover and reset.

Ultimately, training your brain is an investment in *yourself*. It pays dividends in the form of greater focus, steadier emotions, and a sense of control amid life's chaos. As you strengthen your mindfulness habit, you'll likely notice subtle shifts: maybe you don't get as irritated in traffic, or you find it easier to concentrate on that report, or you catch yourself before reacting impulsively in a meeting. Those little shifts are the compound interest on your daily practice. Over months and years, they add up to profound transformation – the kind that people around you will notice, wondering what your "secret" is.

The good news is, this secret is available to everyone. All it takes is a bit of time and consistency, and the willingness to sit quietly and train that most important muscle of all – your mind. So as you move forward, remember to include mental workouts in your routine. Your nervous system will reset, your vagus nerve will thank you, and you'll be building the resilience and clarity needed to truly thrive in work and life. In the quest for peak performance, sharpen your mind as you would sharpen a sword – with daily practice. The results, as science and experience both show, can be life-changing. Now, take a deep breath, carry on with calm focus, and get ready to perform at your best. You've got this!

Chapter 5

Move and Fuel – Exercise and Nutrition for Peak Brain Performance

Body and Brain: An Integrated System

Your brain and body are in constant communication – they don't operate in silos. Every choice you make in physical activity and nutrition sends ripples through this mind-body network, affecting mental clarity, energy levels, and stress resilience. Decades of research confirm that regular exercise yields not just physical fitness but also sharper brain function. Similarly, the food you eat literally becomes fuel for your brain. By optimizing these lifestyle factors, you can create a virtuous cycle: a healthy body supporting a high-performing, resilient mind.

It's easy to think of exercise as something we do for muscles and nutrition as something we do for waistlines. In reality, both are powerful levers for cognitive enhancement and mood regulation. A brisk jog or a set of jumping jacks can clear mental fog and lift your spirits faster than any gadget or nootropic. And the right meal or snack can stabilize your focus when stress threatens to derail you. In this chapter, we'll explore how movement and diet are deeply intertwined with brain performance. You'll discover how working out can act as a stress antidote and brain booster, and how feeding your body well feeds your mind. The goal is to give you practical tools – from scheduling exercise "meetings" with yourself to smart hydration and diet tweaks – so you can thrive under pressure rather than be overwhelmed by it.

Exercise – A Stress Antidote and Brain Booster

You've probably experienced how a good workout can seemingly melt away the day's frustrations. This is not just a mood "illusion" – it's biochemistry in action. Physical activity sets off a cascade of beneficial neurochemical changes that improve your mood, cognition, and stress response. Let's break down why exercise is one of the most powerful (and free!) mental performance enhancers available.

The Neurochemical Rewards of Movement

When you exercise, your body releases a cocktail of chemicals that soothe and sharpen the brain. Chief among these are endorphins, the body's natural painkillers and mood lifters. Endorphins are what generate that post-exercise "glow" or even the legendary "runner's high." They interact with the brain to reduce the perception of pain and trigger positive feelings. At the same time, exercise moderates your stress hormones. In the short term, a workout might spike adrenaline and cortisol (as your body mobilizes energy and responds to exertion), but in the long run regular exercise actually *lowers* baseline cortisol levels and improves your hormonal stress balance. This means that consistent physical activity can make you less prone to feeling chronically stressed or anxious.

Another profound benefit comes from exercise-induced growth factors in the brain. Perhaps the most famous is BDNF (Brain-Derived

Neurotrophic Factor), often nicknamed "Miracle-Gro for the brain" for its role in helping neurons grow and connect. Regular physical exercise has been shown to boost BDNF levels in the brain. Why is that important? Elevated BDNF enhances synaptic plasticity – essentially making it easier for neurons to form new connections. This is associated with better learning, memory retention, and overall cognitive function. In fact, BDNF is so crucial to mental performance that blocking its activity in experiments erases the cognitive benefits of exercise. Higher BDNF levels are also correlated with improved mood and lower rates of depression. Studies have found that optimizing BDNF (through exercise or other means) can lead to greater resilience of brain circuits and alleviation of depressive symptoms. This helps explain why exercise is a potent antidepressant and anxiety-reducer in study after study: it literally nourishes the brain at the cellular level.

Short Bouts for a Quick Brain Boost

When it comes to exercise, you don't need to run marathons to sharpen your mind. Research suggests even *brief* bouts of movement can deliver an immediate cognitive boost. A recent analysis of nearly 20 years of data found that short, vigorous exercise – think cycling sprints, a fast-paced set of burpees, or a quick climb up several flights of stairs – can significantly improve aspects of cognition like memory, attention, and decision-making right after you do it. The effects were strongest for high-intensity activities (like HIIT workouts) and for sessions under 30 minutes. In other words, *quality beats quantity* for acute brain benefits: a hard 10-minute workout can wake up your brain and enhance executive function more than a leisurely 60-minute stroll (though both have their place).

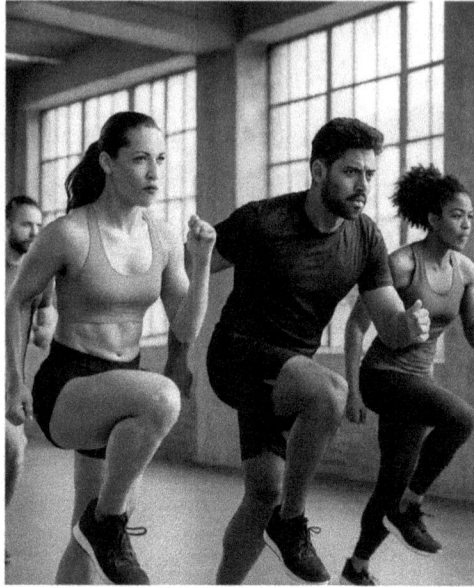

People engaged in a high-intenstty interval training (HilT) workout. Short burst of vigsrous exercise like HilT have been shown to produce immediate improvements in executive function, memory, and other cognitive abilities.

Many high-performers take advantage of these findings by incorporating "exercise snacks" into their workday. Instead of (or in addition to) reaching for another cup of coffee when the afternoon slump hits, they'll do 5 minutes of jumping jacks, push-ups, or a brisk walk around the block. These mini workouts send a rush of blood and oxygen to the brain, along with neurotransmitters that heighten alertness. The result is often a clearer, more energized mind – sometimes *more* effective than caffeine for breaking through fatigue. One reason is that exercise triggers the release of epinephrine and norepinephrine (chemicals related to adrenaline) which sharpen focus and reaction time. So, the next time you feel your brain stalling at 3 PM, try an "exercise snack." A short burst of movement can energize you better than a sugary treat, and without the inevitable crash.

Training Your Stress Resilience

Beyond the immediate chemistry, exercise serves as a training ground for stress resilience. Think about what happens when you push through a tough workout: your heart rate rises, you're breathing hard, your muscles burn, and a voice in your head might be saying "Quit now." In essence, you're voluntarily putting your body into a state of controlled stress. By choosing not to quit and instead persisting through that discomfort, you teach your mind and body a powerful lesson – that *you can handle challenge and come out stronger on the other side.* Over time, this translates into a higher threshold for other types of stress. The research community calls this the "cross-stressor adaptation" hypothesis: the adaptations your body makes to handle exercise stress also help buffer you against mental and emotional stressors. Indeed, physically fit individuals show a more tempered physiological response to psychological stress and are less likely to develop stress-related disorders.

It's no coincidence that many top executives, entrepreneurs, and military leaders are lifelong endurance athletes or martial artists. Engaging in challenging physical pursuits provides a dual benefit: it's an *outlet* to blow off steam and a *practice arena* for mental toughness. Whether it's powering through the last mile of a run or holding that plank pose for an extra 30 seconds, these little victories against discomfort build a reservoir of confidence. The next time you're in a high-pressure meeting or facing a tight deadline, your nervous system remembers: *I've been through intense moments and kept my cool.* In essence, regular exercise raises your stress "tolerance ceiling." You become less likely to be rattled by everyday pressures because your body is used to handling and recovering from stress. One vivid study showed that participants who maintained a regimen of aerobic exercise had significantly blunted cortisol responses to a laboratory stress task compared to sedentary individuals. Simply put, exercise inoculates you against stress – much like a vaccine exposes you to a bit of challenge to protect you from bigger threats down the line.

Making Movement a Daily Habit

Knowing all these benefits is one thing; making exercise a consistent habit is another. The key is to treat exercise like an important meeting with yourself that cannot be missed. Schedule it on your calendar if you must, and protect that time. Consistency matters more than intensity when it comes to stress management and cognitive benefits. A gentle 30-minute walk every day trumps a hardcore workout that you only do once a week. So find activities you truly *enjoy* – enjoyment is the best predictor of consistency. It could be a morning jog listening to your favorite podcast, a lunchtime yoga class to break up your workday, or an evening weightlifting session to blow off steam. It all counts.

Practical tip: Incorporate movement in small ways if you're crunched for time. Walk or bike for errands when possible, take the stairs instead of the elevator, do a few stretches during TV commercial breaks. Even walking the dog counts (and Fido will thank you)! In fact, walking in nature has some special perks. Studies show that walking in green, natural environments can lower cortisol and reduce rumination (repetitive negative thoughts), compared to walking in an urban setting. If you have a park or trail nearby, consider it free medicine for your mind – a brisk walk among the trees can leave you calmer and more focused by the time you return to your desk.

And remember, on days when you truly have *zero* time, doing just a few minutes of movement is far better than doing nothing. Stand up from your desk now and then and do some shoulder rolls, neck stretches, or a quick mobility drill for your back. These micro-breaks keep your body from stiffening up and send a little wake-up call to your brain. The goal is to avoid letting any day become completely sedentary. By prioritizing daily movement, you'll likely find your brain thanking you with sharper focus, better mood, and sounder sleep.

Nutrition – Food for Thought (Literally)

We've all heard the phrase "you are what you eat." From a brain perspective, it's absolutely true: the nutrients (or lack thereof) in your diet have a *direct* impact on cognitive function and emotional balance. The brain is an energy-hungry organ – accounting for about 2% of body weight but consuming roughly 20% of your daily calories. It also has high requirements for certain micronutrients and fatty acids to build neurotransmitters and brain cell membranes. What you feed your body becomes the fuel and raw materials for your brain. So if you're running on caffeine and sugary snacks, your brain might be revving and stalling like an old car with bad gas. In this section, we'll look at how to fuel for peak mental performance. That means maintaining steady blood sugar, staying well-hydrated, and loading up on brain-friendly nutrients, while avoiding the dietary pitfalls that can exacerbate stress and brain fog.

Think of food as a source of stability for mind and body. Ever notice how being overly hungry or dehydrated can make you feel anxious, irritable, or unable to concentrate? Blood sugar swings and even mild dehydration can mimic or worsen stress symptoms. For instance, if you skip meals or eat a high-sugar breakfast, you might experience a spike and crash in glucose that leaves you jittery then exhausted – not ideal for focused work. Even losing 1-2% of your body's water (which can happen after a few hours of intense work without drinking) has been shown to impair concentration and elevate cortisol (the stress hormone). On the flip side, a balanced diet rich in whole foods supplies steady energy and essential nutrients, keeping your brain on an even keel during the day's challenges. Let's break down some core nutrition principles and tips for high performance living:

Stable Energy for a Sharp Brain

One of the best things you can do for your brain is to maintain stable blood sugar levels. Large swings – either too high or too low – can cause that infamous "brain fog" or sudden crashes in energy. Start by *prioritizing protein*, especially in the morning. Don't skip protein at breakfast. While a glazed pastry or bowl of sugary cereal may give you a quick rush, it's likely to spike your blood glucose and then send it plummeting a couple hours later. The result? Fatigue, irritability, and difficulty concentrating once the "sugar crash" hits. In contrast, a breakfast with sufficient protein and healthy fats (think eggs with avocado, Greek yogurt with nuts, or a protein smoothie with berries and spinach) leads to a slower, steadier release of glucose. Protein foods provide amino acids like tyrosine and tryptophan, which are the building blocks for key neurotransmitters such as dopamine and serotonin. Dopamine, made from tyrosine, is crucial for motivation and focus, while serotonin (from tryptophan) regulates mood and calm. By including protein in your morning meal, you give your brain the raw materials to synthesize these chemicals, setting you up for sustained alertness and a balanced mood. Many people report that when they switch from a carb-heavy breakfast (e.g. a muffin or bagel) to a protein-rich one, they experience far less mid-morning slump and cravings.

Equally important is not going too long without eating during the day. If you've ever been *hangry* (hungry-angry), you know how low blood sugar can manifest as anxiety or short-temperedness. Physiologically, when your blood sugar drops too low, the body perceives it as a stressor and pumps out adrenaline and cortisol to compensate. This is why you might feel shaky or on edge when extremely hungry – your body is literally in a mini fight-or-flight mode due to lack of fuel. Avoid that scenario by having balanced meals and snacks at regular intervals. A good rule of thumb is to include some protein, fiber (vegetables or whole grains), and healthy fat in each meal. The combination of these macronutrients slows digestion and provides a sustained energy release, preventing wild swings in blood glucose.

Stay hydrated as part of your energy management. The brain is about 75% water, and even mild dehydration can cause headaches, poor concentration, and heightened perception of stress. In fact, one study found that men who were ~1.5% dehydrated (a relatively small deficit) showed measurable impairments in memory and increases in anxiety/tension. Aim to drink water regularly throughout the day. Keep a water bottle at your desk as a visual reminder. If plain water bores you, jazz it up with a squeeze of lemon or a few mint leaves, or sip herbal teas. A smart habit is to start your morning with a large glass of water (you've been fasting all night, after all). Some experts suggest adding a pinch of sea salt and a squeeze of lemon to that first glass – the electrolytes help rehydrate you faster, and the ritual can boost your alertness even before the caffeine kicks in.

Caffeine: Friend or Foe?

Speaking of caffeine, it's the world's most widely used stimulant, and it can be a double-edged sword for high performance. In moderation, caffeine enhances alertness, mood, and even aspects of cognitive function like reaction time and vigilance. A cup of coffee or tea in the morning can help shake off grogginess and get your brain into gear. Caffeine works primarily by blocking adenosine receptors in the brain (adenosine is a chemical that builds up to signal fatigue), essentially putting a brake on the sleepiness signal. It also triggers the release of dopamine and adrenaline, which can improve focus and energy. So yes, that morning brew can be genuinely helpful for mental acuity.

However, trouble arises when we overdo it or mistime it. Too much caffeine can make you jittery, anxious, and can raise your heart rate – basically mirroring the physical sensations of stress. There's also a genetic component: some people are slow caffeine metabolizers and are more sensitive to its effects. Research has confirmed that high doses of caffeine (especially above ~400 mg, or around 4 strong cups of coffee per day) are linked to increased anxiety levels. If you've ever had one espresso too many and felt your mind race or your hands tremble, you've experienced this. Additionally, consuming caffeine too late in the day can sabotage your sleep. Caffeine has a half-life of about 5-6 hours in most people, meaning if you drink a big coffee at 4 p.m., about half of that caffeine could still be in your system by 10 p.m. It's no surprise that caffeine can reduce sleep quality and duration. And poor sleep then creates a vicious cycle – you wake up tired, reaching for even more caffeine to compensate.

So how do we get the benefits of caffeine while minimizing downsides? Strategic use. Many sleep and performance experts (such as Dr. Andrew Huberman and others) suggest delaying your first caffeine dose to 60–90 minutes after waking. The reasoning is that your cortisol naturally peaks in the first hour of waking – helping you feel alert. If you flood your system with caffeine at the same time, you may crash harder when both the caffeine and cortisol wear off around mid-morning. By waiting an hour or so, you let cortisol do its job, then use caffeine as a *secondary boost*. This practice can also extend the effectiveness of your caffeine high into late morning. Another tip: try to cut off caffeine at least 8 hours before bedtime. If you go to bed at 11 p.m., that means no caffeine after ~3 p.m. (earlier if you're especially caffeine-sensitive). This gives your body time to metabolize most of it so it doesn't interfere with deep sleep. Remember, even if you can *fall* asleep after a late coffee, caffeine can disrupt the *quality* of your sleep (reducing restorative deep sleep), and you might wake up less refreshed.

Consider experimenting with green tea or adding L-theanine alongside your caffeine. Green tea naturally contains the amino acid *L-theanine*, which promotes a calm, focused mental state. L-theanine increases alpha brain waves (associated with relaxed alertness) and can boost levels of GABA and dopamine, leading to reduced anxiety and improved concentration. When taken with caffeine, L-theanine has been found to smooth out the jitters and enhance cognitive performance more than caffeine alone. This combination – often a 2:1 ratio of L-theanine (in mg) to caffeine – is popular among professionals and gamers who want prolonged focus without the frazzle. You can get this effect by simply drinking green tea (which has less caffeine than coffee plus L-theanine), or by taking an L-theanine supplement with your coffee. Either way, the result is often a steadier, calmer alertness. Of course, individual responses vary, so pay attention to how you feel and adjust accordingly.

Nutrients for Cognitive Edge

Fueling a high-performance brain isn't just about macronutrients and stimulants; it's also about the micronutrients and specific fats that directly support brain structure and function. Two big dietary rock stars for the brain are omega-3 fatty acids and antioxidant-rich plant foods (like leafy greens and berries).

Omega-3 fats, particularly DHA and EPA (found in fatty fish like salmon, sardines, as well as walnuts and flaxseeds in the form of ALA), are crucial for the brain. DHA is a major structural fat in brain cell membranes; it makes up a large portion of the gray matter. Having ample DHA is associated with better cell communication and reduced inflammation in the brain. Research has shown that consuming omega-3s can *improve learning, memory and overall cognitive well-being*, and even increase blood flow in the brain. Omega-3s are also well-known to have anti-inflammatory effects. Since chronic inflammation can exacerbate stress and is linked to mood disorders, keeping inflammation in check is important for mental resilience. One remarkable study found that medical students who took omega-3 supplements during a stressful exam period had significantly lower inflammation markers and experienced a 20% reduction in anxiety symptoms compared to a placebo group. It's as if omega-3s help put out some of the "fire" that stress ignites in the body. To get more of these beneficial fats, aim to include fatty fish in your diet a couple of times a week or consider a quality fish oil supplement if needed (especially if you follow a vegetarian diet). Plant sources like chia seeds, flax, and walnuts are great too – though they provide ALA which the body partially converts to DHA/EPA.

Equally important are leafy greens and colorful fruits – essentially, high-antioxidant foods. Oxidative stress (caused by free radicals) is a byproduct of both normal metabolism and stress, and it can damage cells over time, including brain cells. Antioxidants are like rust-proofing for your brain: they neutralize those free radicals. Leafy greens such as spinach, kale, collards, and broccoli are packed with vitamins (like vitamin K, folate) and carotenoids (like lutein and beta-carotene) that have been linked to slower cognitive decline. In one long-term study, older adults who consumed at least one serving of leafy greens a day had the cognitive abilities of people 11 years younger than their actual age, compared to those who rarely ate greens. The likely reason is a mix of nutrients that protect the brain. For example, lutein (abundant in spinach and kale) accumulates in neural tissue and is thought to improve processing speed and memory.

Beyond greens, "eat the rainbow" of fruits and veggies to cover a spectrum of antioxidants. Berries (blueberries, strawberries, blackberries) are rich in flavonoids that have been shown to improve communication between brain cells and reduce cognitive aging. In fact, blueberries are so renowned for brain health that they're nicknamed "brainberries" by some scientists. Citrus fruits, cherries, and dark chocolate (yes, in moderation, dark chocolate's cocoa flavanols count too) also contribute antioxidant compounds. These foods not only fight oxidative stress but often reduce inflammation as well, creating a favorable environment for your brain to function under pressure. Think of a dish like a salmon and spinach salad with colorful peppers and walnuts – it's a stress-fighting, brain-boosting powerhouse meal, providing omega-3s, antioxidants, fiber, and protein all in one.

Lastly, don't forget about micronutrients like magnesium, B-vitamins, and zinc. These often act as cofactors in neurotransmitter production and energy metabolism in the brain. For instance, magnesium has a calming effect on the nervous system (it helps regulate neurotransmitters and the HPA axis that controls stress hormones). Many adults don't get enough magnesium from diet alone (it's found in nuts, seeds, leafy greens, beans), so ensuring you have magnesium-rich foods can help with relaxation and sleep quality. If you struggle with tense muscles or anxiety, it might be worth discussing with your doctor whether a magnesium supplement (often magnesium glycinate for calming benefits) could be helpful. Similarly, B-vitamins (like B6, B12, folate) are crucial for mood regulation and cognitive function – they help in the synthesis of serotonin, dopamine, and also support healthy homocysteine levels (elevated homocysteine is linked to cognitive decline). A well-rounded diet with whole grains, proteins, and vegetables typically provides these, but during periods of intense stress your body may use up certain nutrients faster. That's why a multi-vitamin or specific supplements are sometimes considered by high-performers as an insurance policy. Which brings us to a final point on supplements.

Smart Supplementation (with Caution)

In the quest for peak performance, some individuals experiment with adaptogens and nootropics – herbs or compounds that purportedly help the body adapt to stress or enhance cognitive function. One popular adaptogenic herb is Ashwagandha (Withania somnifera), used for centuries in Ayurvedic medicine. Modern research is lending credibility to its stress-relieving reputation. For example, a recent meta-analysis of 9 randomized trials (involving 558 people) found that Ashwagandha supplementation was associated with significantly *lower* stress and anxiety scores, and notably *reduced cortisol levels*, compared to placebo. Participants taking Ashwagandha had improved outcomes on stress questionnaires and a roughly 30% reduction in morning cortisol on average, which is quite remarkable. These results suggest Ashwagandha can help temper the physiological stress response and improve subjective well-being under stress. It's no magic cure-all, but for some it serves as a helpful adjunct to lifestyle measures.

Another supplement often mentioned for stress and relaxation is Magnesium – as noted, it's involved in calming the nervous system and many people have suboptimal intake. Some studies have found that magnesium supplementation can modestly reduce anxiety and improve sleep, particularly in individuals who are deficient. Forms like magnesium glycinate or magnesium threonate are typically used for mental health benefits. L-theanine, which we discussed earlier, is also available as a supplement (often in the 100-200 mg range) to promote relaxation without sedation.

Caution: While supplements can be beneficial, they are highly individual in their effects and are not rigorously regulated like pharmaceuticals. Quality and dosage matter. It's wise to consult with a healthcare professional before starting any new supplement, especially if you take medications (since even natural compounds can have interactions). Adaptogens like Ashwagandha are generally well-tolerated, but they may not be suitable for everyone (for instance, those with autoimmune conditions or thyroid issues should use caution, as some evidence suggests Ashwagandha can affect thyroid hormones). The same goes for high doses of magnesium (too much can cause digestive upset) or any nootropic compound – more isn't always better. Think of supplements as the "cherry on top" of your stress-management and performance toolkit. The foundation should still be solid nutrition, exercise, sleep, and other lifestyle practices. No pill or powder can compensate for a poor diet or chronic sleep deprivation in the long run.

The Synergy of Move and Fuel: Thriving Under Pressure

We've explored exercise and nutrition separately, but it's worth emphasizing how powerful they are together. These are not isolated domains; they reinforce each other in a positive feedback loop. When you eat well, you have more energy and motivation to exercise. When you exercise regularly, you tend to make better food choices (in part because your body starts craving quality fuel). This synergy is a secret sauce for peak performance.

Consider a typical afternoon crisis: You've been working hard all day, stress is building, and you feel an energy lull around 3–4 PM. Your brain starts screaming for a quick reward – perhaps a candy bar or some chips from the vending machine. That sugar rush sounds tempting as a quick fix for your flagging focus. This is the perfect moment to leverage move *and* fuel instead of reaching for junk. First, get moving for 10 minutes. Step outside if you can and take a brisk walk, or do a mini workout in your office or living room (a set of bodyweight squats or a quick yoga flow). This physical activity will lower your stress hormones (clearing out some of that cortisol and adrenaline) and boost endorphins, likely improving your mood and clearing the mental cobwebs. Movement also increases blood circulation to the brain, giving you a hit of oxygen and nutrients right when you need it.

After the movement break, have a smart snack. Instead of a candy bar (which would spike your blood sugar and then send it crashing, exacerbating fatigue), choose something with protein and/or healthy fat to stabilize you. For example, a handful of almonds or walnuts, a piece of fruit with a few slices of cheese, or some Greek yogurt with berries. The walk plus the nutritious snack work in tandem: the walk blunts the stress and re-energizes your mind, and the snack replenishes your brain's fuel supply steadily without a crash. By 4 PM, you've now turned what could have been a downward spiral into a second wind of productivity – all without the guilt or grogginess that a junk-food binge would have caused.

Another way the "move and fuel" combo plays out is in sleep quality, which is foundational for resilience. Exercise (especially when done earlier in the day) can significantly improve sleep depth and duration. Eating a balanced diet, and not too late at night, also sets the stage for good sleep. In turn, quality sleep balances hormones like cortisol and hunger hormones, making it easier to stick to exercise and healthy eating the next day. You can see how each pillar supports the others.

As we wrap up, remember this overarching theme: *your body is the vehicle that carries your brain.* Treat your body well, and your mind will reap the benefits – from sharper focus and creativity to a calmer baseline under stress. In the heat of a busy work project or life challenge, it's easy to neglect exercise or grab convenient but poor fuel. But those are the times when staying on track with movement and nutrition pays the greatest dividends. Even just a quick stretch and a glass of water can reset your stress response in the middle of chaos. Over time, these habits build a sort of physical and mental armor. You become the person who doesn't crumble when deadlines loom or when multiple demands pile up – instead, you have energy in reserve and a mind that stays clear under pressure.

Chapter 5 Key Takeaways (Move and Fuel for Peak Brain Performance):

- **Exercise is a Cognitive Enhancer:** Regular physical activity triggers biochemical changes that improve mood and brain function. It releases endorphins (boosting pleasure, reducing pain) and increases BDNF, a growth factor that strengthens neural connections for better memory and learning. Consistent exercise also lowers chronic stress hormone levels and can alleviate symptoms of anxiety and depression over time. It's like a natural antidepressant and focus booster rolled into one.

- **Even Short Workouts Count:** You don't need hours at the gym to get brain benefits. Brief bursts of vigorous exercise (10–20 minutes of HIIT or a fast run) can immediately sharpen your attention and executive function by increasing blood flow and neurotransmitters in the brain. Using "exercise snacks" – short movement breaks during your day – is an effective strategy to re-energize during slumps.

- **Build Stress Resilience Through Movement:** Pushing through physical challenges teaches your body and brain to handle stress better. Regular exercise raises your threshold for stress, making you less reactive to everyday pressures. Fitter individuals have been shown to have more muted physiological responses to stressors. In essence, exercise is like a vaccine that exposes you to controlled stress to fortify your resilience.

- **Nutrition Fuels Mental Performance:** The brain consumes ~20% of your calories, so stable energy intake is crucial. Emphasize protein and fiber-rich foods to avoid blood sugar crashes that can cause fatigue and irritability. Stay hydrated, since even mild dehydration can impair cognition and mood. A well-fed brain (with steady glucose, adequate protein, and micronutrients) will concentrate longer and remain steadier under strain.

- **Be Strategic with Stimulants:** Caffeine can boost alertness and mood in moderate doses, but use it wisely. Have your first coffee about 60–90 minutes after waking (to ride the natural cortisol wave) and cut off caffeine by early afternoon to protect sleep quality. Total intake above 400 mg can increase anxiety in many people. Consider green tea or adding L-theanine to coffee for a calmer focus boost.

- **Omega-3s and Greens Are Brain Food:** Foods rich in omega-3 fatty acids (like salmon, sardines, flaxseed, walnuts) provide DHA for brain cell structure and have anti-inflammatory effects that support mood and cognitive health. Studies show omega-3 intake is linked to improved learning, memory, and even reduced anxiety under stress. Likewise, leafy greens and colorful fruits/veggies supply antioxidants that protect the brain from oxidative stress and aging, contributing to better mental function over time. A diet high in these foods is associated with a more resilient brain.

- **Consider Supplements Carefully:** Certain supplements like *Ashwagandha* (an adaptogenic herb) have evidence for reducing stress and cortisol, and *Magnesium* can support relaxation and sleep, but they should complement – not replace – healthy lifestyle habits. Always research quality and consult a professional if in doubt. Supplements can be helpful tools, but individual responses vary, and they work best on top of a solid foundation of good diet and exercise.

By moving your body regularly and fueling it with intention, you create optimal conditions for your brain to excel. It's all connected: a workout isn't just a treat for your muscles, it's a gift to your mind; a healthy meal isn't just nourishment for your body, it's power for your neurons. Make the choice, day by day, to prioritize these habits. In doing so, you'll build the energy, focus, and stress resilience that set you up for success in work and life – a true "nervous system reset" whenever you need it.

Chapter 6

The Flow of Work – Finding Focus and Productivity without Burning Out

We've spent time on how to care for your body and mind outside of work – now it's time to optimize how you work itself. Peak performance isn't a simple matter of raw hours logged. It depends more on the quality of your attention and finding the right balance between exertion and rest. Many of us fall into the trap of equating "busyness" with productivity, juggling a dozen tasks at once and grinding for hours without a break. It may *feel* like you're getting a lot done, but neuroscience and psychology research suggest a smarter approach: alternate periods of intense, focused work with short breaks, and cultivate a mental state of flow. Paradoxically, this approach lets you accomplish more in less time – and with less mental exhaustion – than the frantic, non-stop hustle.

The Myth of Multitasking: Why One Thing at a Time Beats Task Switching

Let's burst a common bubble: multitasking. Despite how it appears, our brains are not actually doing two things at once; they're rapidly *switching* focus from one thing to another. And that switching carries a cost. Studies show that frequent task-switching can slash productivity by up to 40% and increase the likelihood of errors. In practical terms, every time you bounce between an email and a report, or between five different browser tabs, your brain has to re-orient itself. This "switching tax" leaves you feeling frazzled and mentally drained as the day wears on. In fact, research by psychologist David Meyer found that even brief mental blocks created by shifting between tasks can cost a significant chunk of your productive time.

Multitasking doesn't just hamper efficiency – it also spikes stress. Each little switch triggers a mild stress response as your brain scrambles to refocus. As one article vividly put it, multitasking *"hamstrings productivity by as much as 40 percent… and even dings your IQ"*. Indeed, in one experiment, people who multitasked during cognitive tasks experienced IQ score drops equivalent to missing a full night of sleep. So if you've ever felt scatter-brained after trying to do too many things at once, you're not imagining it – you literally can become less sharp. Moreover, once you do get pulled off track, it can take a while to regain full focus. A University of California–Irvine study famously found it takes about 23 minutes on average to get back to a task after an interruption. Think about that – a single "quick check" of email or a phone notification can potentially sap nearly half an hour of productive time as you ramp back up.

The take-home message is crystal clear: you'll perform better and feel better if you single-task. In practice, this means giving your full attention to one thing at a time – whether it's writing a report, having a meeting, or even reading your emails – and resisting the urge to simultaneously handle unrelated tasks. By batching and focusing, you'll complete each item more efficiently than if you try to do them all in parallel. Give yourself permission to ignore the myriad other things vying for your attention until you finish the task at hand. You may worry that you'll be less responsive or slower, but the reality is that you'll get more done *overall*. And as we'll explore, there are ways to manage expectations and communication so that single-tasking is both feasible and respected in your workplace.

Embrace Deep Work and Flow for Peak Performance

So what should replace multitasking? The answer is deep, focused work – the kind that can lead to the highly productive mental state known as flow. *Flow* is that coveted state described by psychologist Mihály Csíkszentmihályi, where you become fully absorbed in an activity, time seems to fly, and you perform at your best. In a flow state, you aren't anxious or bored; you're challenged *just* the right amount relative to your skill level, leading to a feeling of energized focus and effortless action. Think of times when you've been "in the zone" – maybe you were coding for hours or absorbed in a creative project, and when you finally looked up, you were astonished to see how much time had passed. That's flow.

Achieving flow at work might sound mystical, but research has uncovered practical conditions that encourage it. Csíkszentmihályi's studies found that having clear goals and unbroken focus are key conditions for flow. In other words, you should know what you're trying to accomplish and have the freedom to concentrate deeply without interruptions. This aligns perfectly with the concept of "deep work," popularized by author Cal Newport. Deep work means carving out uninterrupted blocks of time to push your cognitive limits on meaningful tasks, free from distractions. It's the opposite of the fragmented, notification-driven mode of work that is so common today.

To practice deep work, Newport recommends proactively blocking off chunks of time and creating an environment that shields you from interruption. That means muting your phone, shutting down email and chat apps, and secluding yourself if possible during those focus periods. You might put on noise-cancelling headphones or find a quiet room. Let colleagues know you'll be in "focus mode" for a while. These actions signal to both yourself and others that you are doing valued, high-level work that deserves protection. It may feel odd at first to be less available moment-to-moment, but this is exactly how top performers produce high-quality output. They devote fully present attention to the task at hand.

Flow also requires that the task itself is neither too easy (leading to boredom) nor too hard (leading to anxiety). Whenever possible, match your tasks to your skill level, upping the challenge as your skills improve. Break a big project into smaller milestones so that you always have a clear, achievable goal in front of you. Csíkszentmihályi noted that flow often occurs when one's skills are just sufficient to meet a challenging goal, in a situation that provides immediate feedback on performance. In a work context, that might mean setting a specific target for a focus session ("I'm going to draft the first section of this report in the next 90 minutes") and then being able to see progress at the end of that session. Each mini-achievement provides feedback and a sense of progress, which can encourage the flow state to continue.

Cultivating flow and deep work is like training a muscle – it gets stronger with practice. Initially, you might find it hard to concentrate deeply for more than 15 or 20 minutes if you're used to constant distraction. That's okay. Start small, and gradually extend your focus sessions. Over time, as your brain adapts, you'll find it easier to drop into deep focus and maybe even experience that blissful immersion of flow on a regular basis. The payoff is huge: not only will you get more done, but you'll likely find the work itself more rewarding and less stressful when you're fully engaged. As Csíkszentmihályi showed, deep focus can even boost happiness and fulfillment, turning work into a source of genuine satisfaction.

Strategies to Engineer Focus and Flow in Your Workday

It's one thing to talk about focus and flow in theory, but how do you actually create these conditions in the middle of a busy workday? Here are several concrete strategies to help you work smarter:

- **Time Blocking for Deep Work:** Proactively schedule dedicated blocks on your calendar for high-priority tasks, and treat them as you would an important meeting or appointment. For example, you might block out 9–11 AM for writing or brainstorming when you know your energy is high. During these blocks, eliminate distractions – put your phone on Do Not Disturb, close your email and chat apps, and if possible, shut your door or put on headphones to signal you're in focus mode. You might even put a note on your status or desk saying "Focus Time – back at 11." By creating this protected bubble for deep work, you give your brain the chance to fully engage with one task. You're effectively saying: "This is important, and everything else can wait." People who adopt time blocking often find that tasks which used to stretch out all day get done much faster in a pressure-free, uninterrupted hour. Cal Newport and others attest that consistently scheduling these blocks – even just a couple of hours a day – can dramatically increase your productive output. It may require some communication and discipline (for instance, letting colleagues know why you're unavailable for a period), but the payoff is worth it when you see how much quality work you produce in those sacred focus blocks.

- **Leverage Breaks as a Performance Tool, Not a Waste of Time:** It might feel counterintuitive, but taking short breaks can actually *improve* your overall productivity and focus. Research from the University of Illinois found that even very brief mental breaks can dramatically improve focus and prevent performance declines over long tasks. In that study, people who took a couple of one-minute breaks during a 50-minute task maintained their level of performance, while those who worked straight through saw their performance steadily drop over time. The brain is wired to detect and respond to change; when stimulation is constant and unvarying, our brains start to tune it out. In practical terms, if you stare at a spreadsheet or a report for too long without pause, your attention may flatline. Stepping away for even 5 minutes resets this mechanism and can refresh your concentration for the next round of work. This is the idea behind popular techniques like the *Pomodoro method*, where you work for about 25 minutes, then take a 5-minute break, and repeat. During your breaks, do something different: stand up and stretch, grab a glass of water, look out a window, or walk around the office. Give your eyes a rest from the screen. These micro-breaks are not "lost" time – they are investments in sustaining high-quality focus. In fact, you'll likely get that time back through faster, sharper work when you resume. As one researcher put it, *"Brief mental breaks will actually help you stay focused on your task!"*. The key is to truly disconnect for a few minutes – don't jump to a different work task or social media (which only keeps your brain in a state of frenetic input). Let your mind reset.

- **Prioritize Ruthlessly and Delegate When Possible:** A common cause of burnout is trying to do everything yourself. High performers can be prone to perfectionism and the belief that if they want something done right, they have to do it all. But part of working smarter is ruthless prioritization of where you invest your energy. Each day, identify your "MITs" – your Most Important Tasks – ideally the top two or three tasks that will have the highest impact on your goals. Plan to tackle those first, during the time of day when you have the most energy (more on energy cycles shortly). Less critical tasks can be scheduled for later, delegated to others, or sometimes dropped entirely. Remember the 80/20 rule (Pareto principle): often 20% of tasks yield 80% of the results. If you can pinpoint which tasks are in that vital 20%, you can focus on them and avoid getting lost perfecting the trivial many. For example, if responding to routine emails or formatting a document isn't moving the needle on your big goals, consider whether you can do it later in a low-energy moment or hand it off to an assistant or colleague. This also means learning to say "no" or "not now" to tasks and meetings that aren't truly necessary. It can be uncomfortable, especially if you're used to being a go-to person, but it's critical for preventing overload. By being selective about your commitments, you preserve your mental bandwidth for the work that really matters. This approach isn't just about personal productivity, either – it often leads to better results for your team or business because you're ensuring that talent and time are applied where they have the most impact. In sum, *don't burn yourself out trying to chase a 5% improvement on something unimportant, while the big stuff languishes.* Do the important 20% exceptionally well and let the rest follow.

- **Design Your Work for Flow (as much as possible):** Whenever you have latitude, structure your work environment and schedule to increase autonomy and meaning. Flow tends to thrive when you have some control over *how* you do a task and when you can connect the task to a meaningful purpose. If you're in a leadership position, consider giving your team members regular chunks of time with no meetings or interruptions, so they can dive deep into their projects. (Some forward-thinking companies have instituted "meeting-free days" for this purpose – with impressive results. In one study, companies that introduced just two meeting-free days a week saw productivity rise by over 70%, as employees felt more empowered to manage their time and experienced less stress.) If you're an individual contributor and your calendar is a sea of meetings, see if you can consolidate or eliminate any that aren't absolutely necessary. Perhaps propose that your team experiment with a meeting-free afternoon each week, or at least stack meetings back-to-back in parts of the day so that you have other hours completely open. Fewer interruptions = more opportunities for flow. Science backs this up: when people have greater autonomy over their work – the freedom to choose what to work on and how to do it – they tend to be more productive *and* more satisfied. So, whenever possible, arrange your workflow to give yourself that autonomy. This might mean negotiating deadlines so you can work in focused bursts, or setting up your workspace to minimize random drop-ins (maybe wearing headphones as a do-not-disturb signal or working from home/library for deep work stints if your office allows it). Additionally, try to find meaning in your tasks. It's easier to enter flow when you value the task's purpose. Sometimes reframing a task in terms of the bigger picture ("answering these support tickets helps our customers succeed, which is why we're here") can boost engagement. Finally, break big projects into clear milestones or sub-goals. Each milestone can serve as a mini goalpost that provides a sense of progress and feedback, which encourages flow by signaling to your brain that you're on the right track. Completing a milestone gives you a little dopamine hit of accomplishment and motivates you to tackle the next one.

Case Study: Batching Emails – How One Manager Regained Hours of Focus

To illustrate these principles, let's look at a typical scenario. Consider a mid-level manager – we'll call him Jason – who used to keep his email inbox open all day. Jason prided himself on being responsive; if an email came in, he would jump on it within minutes. He believed this made him a good team player and efficient worker. But the reality was that his day was getting shredded by constant context switching. Every few minutes, a new message would steal his attention, forcing his brain to switch gears. He'd start working on a report, then *ping!* an email about an unrelated issue would pop up, and he'd feel obliged to answer. By the time he returned to the report, he had lost momentum (remember that 23-minute recovery time). The result: Jason would reach the end of a busy day feeling like he hadn't accomplished much *real* work, and he often had to stay late to finish tasks in the quiet evening hours.

After learning about the deep work concept, Jason decided to experiment with a new system: checking email only at two scheduled times per day, say at 11:00am and 4:00pm, and closing his email program outside those windows. He communicated to colleagues that he might not respond immediately to emails because he was implementing some "focus times" to get important work done, but he assured them he'd still answer by end of day. At first, he felt anxious – what if something urgent came up and he missed it by not checking constantly? But soon he realized that nothing was on fire; the world didn't end if he responded in a few hours instead of a few minutes. In fact, to his surprise, his productivity in project work skyrocketed. By protecting a few longer spans for focused work (in which he closed Outlook, silenced his phone, and even put a "Do Not Disturb – in Focus Mode until 11am" note on Slack), he found he could accomplish in two hours what used to take an entire fragmented day. He also discovered that when he batched his email responses at those scheduled times, he handled them more efficiently. Instead of drafting one email, then switching to another task, then back to another email, he would go through all his new emails in one go. He became quicker at processing them because his brain was in "email mode" for that block of time.

The overall effect? Jason cut his late-evening catch-up work in half. He went home earlier, feeling less mentally fried. And importantly, nothing blew up in the interim. By being a bit less available moment-to-moment, he was actually *more effective overall*. He did have to gently train some colleagues out of the expectation of an immediate reply (which he handled by using an email auto-reply during focus blocks, or a polite note in his signature about his response times). But over a short period, everyone adapted. They even respected him more for managing his time and priorities well. This case illustrates a powerful point: much of the "urgency" that drives us to multitask or constantly check in is self-imposed. If you set reasonable boundaries (and of course, clear it with your team or boss as needed), you often find that you can create space for deep work without derailing collaboration. In fact, you might inspire others to do the same. Jason's story is a testament to how being less reactive and more intentional with your attention can dramatically improve productivity and reduce burnout.

Finding Your Personal Work Rhythm

Another crucial aspect of working smarter is to find your natural concentration rhythm and work *with* it rather than against it. Everyone's energy and focus levels cycle throughout the day. Some people are at their mental peak first thing in the morning – the classic "early birds" who do their best thinking at dawn. Others are night owls who hit their creative stride after most of the office has gone home. Many of us have a common *mid-afternoon slump* where focus dips (often sometime between 2–4 PM). These patterns are largely driven by your circadian rhythm – the internal biological clock that influences your sleep-wake cycle and energy levels. It's normal, for instance, to feel a bit sluggish after lunch as part of the body's natural circadian schedule. One scientific explanation is that there is a smaller secondary wave of sleepiness roughly 12 hours after the big nightly one, which for most people falls in the early-to-mid afternoon. Combine that with a heavy lunch or a stuffy office, and you have the recipe for drowsy, unfocused hours.

The key is to pay attention to your own patterns. Start observing over a week or two: when do you naturally feel most alert, energetic, and able to tackle complex work? When do you feel the most drained or distracted? Once you have a sense, try to align your task schedule with your biological prime times. For example, if you discover you're mentally sharp in the morning, plan to do your high-concentration tasks (writing, analysis, strategic planning – whatever requires brainpower) in that window. Protect it as your deep work time. Conversely, if you know that every day around 3 PM you hit a wall, don't schedule intensive work then if you can help it. Use that low-energy time for less demanding activities: clearing your inbox (if it doesn't require heavy thinking), doing routine admin or paperwork, or even taking a genuine break to recharge. A short power nap (20 minutes), a walk outside for some fresh air and sunlight, or a meditation session can work wonders to lift you out of an afternoon funk. In fact, studies show a 20–30 minute nap can boost alertness and mood, making you more effective for the remainder of the day.

If napping isn't feasible, simply stepping away from your work for a bit can help. Even a cup of tea and a stretch, or a chat with a coworker, can reset your energy. The idea is not to *fight* your fatigue with sheer willpower (and gallons of coffee) but to flow with it – do something different until your energy naturally rebounds. Similarly, if you're one of those late-night geniuses who suddenly gets inspired at 10 PM, consider if there's flexibility in your schedule to accommodate that – maybe you shift some work to the evening (if your life allows) and start a bit later the next day. Not everyone has complete control over their work hours, but within the constraints you *do* have, you can often tweak things. Even scheduling a creative task you enjoy during a usual low point can sometimes counteract the slump because it engages you in a different way.

By aligning work tasks with your biological prime times, you'll be working with the grain of your brain's natural tendencies. You'll likely find that tasks feel easier and you get into flow more readily when timing is right. In contrast, forcing yourself to do your hardest work at a time when your brain is typically semi-shutdown (for example, demanding creativity at 3 PM if that's your low point, or expecting yourself to write brilliantly late at night when you're a morning person) is like swimming upstream. Whenever possible, do the hardest work when you feel most alert and creative, and do lighter work when you tend to feel a bit duller. Over the long run, this strategy keeps your productivity more consistent and prevents the frustration of spinning your wheels during an "off" period.

Celebrate Small Wins to Sustain Motivation

Finally, let's talk about maintaining your motivation and momentum over the long term. One of the most satisfying aspects of reaching a flow state or completing a deep work session is the feeling of accomplishment that comes with it. You've probably experienced that little rush when you finish a major section of a project or solve a thorny problem – it's energizing. It turns out that *acknowledging these small wins* is more than just a nice feeling; it can train your brain to be even more productive and focused in the future. Psychologists Teresa Amabile and Steven Kramer, who studied hundreds of employees through daily work diaries, coined the term "the progress principle." It means that making progress – even small, incremental progress – on meaningful work is one of the biggest boosters of mood and motivation during a workday. In fact, their research showed that these *tiny victories* can dramatically increase people's engagement and drive at work.

What does this mean for you? It means that you should celebrate small wins and consciously log your progress. When you finish a focus block or hit a milestone, take a brief moment to acknowledge it. This could be as simple as giving yourself a mental high-five ("That presentation outline is done – nice!") or jotting down a note in a work journal about what you achieved today. Some people like to keep a "done list" in addition to their to-do list, where they write down things they completed – this provides a tangible record of progress. These positive reinforcements aren't merely feel-good gimmicks; they actually train your brain to seek more flow experiences. By rewarding yourself (even with just praise or a short break) for a state of deep focus and completion, you create a positive feedback loop. Your brain learns that *this* is the kind of work that brings satisfaction, which can make it easier to start the next task and enter flow again. Over time, this habit builds a mindset where progress itself becomes motivating. Instead of always chasing the next big accomplishment or only feeling satisfied when a project is 100% complete, you'll gain satisfaction from the day-to-day victories that move you forward. This reduces the chance of burnout because you're not perpetually feeling "behind" or overwhelmed – you have evidence each day that you've achieved something, and that boosts your confidence and resilience.

On tough days when motivation is lacking, looking back at a log of small wins ("Last week I wrote five pages, fixed two bugs in the code, and had a great client call") can remind you that *progress is being made*, even if the ultimate goal is still on the horizon. It can rekindle your energy to keep going. In essence, by celebrating small wins, you nurture an inner sense of progress and competence, which fuels a sustainable cycle of productivity.

In Summary: Work Smarter to Perform Better (Without Burning Out)

Working smarter – not just harder – comes down to structuring your day and environment to maximize quality focus, while also giving yourself permission to rest so that you can re-focus effectively. By single-tasking instead of multitasking, you eliminate the productivity losses and stress of constant context-switching. By carving out periods of deep work and cultivating flow, you tap into your brain's fullest potential and creativity, rather than skimming the surface with divided attention. By alternating intensive focus with brief breaks, you respect the way your brain operates and prevent burnout before it starts. You prioritize what truly matters and let go of or delegate the rest, ensuring your energy is spent where it counts most. You tweak your schedule to fit your natural rhythms, rather than fighting against your biological clock. And you take time to acknowledge progress, fueling your motivation with each small success.

The result of these practices is a calmer, more controlled sense of productivity. Instead of that frantic "I'm always behind" feeling, you end the day knowing exactly what you accomplished. You'll likely find you get more done in a day than before, yet have more gas left in the tank by evening. Your nervous system, including that vagus nerve we've talked about elsewhere in this book, thrives on this balanced approach – intense engagement coupled with deliberate recovery. In the long run, this means better performance at work *and* more energy for life outside of work. You're not just optimizing work for work's sake; you're creating a sustainable way to excel in your career without sacrificing your health or happiness. By harnessing the science of focus and flow, you truly set yourself up for peak performance in work and life, on your own terms. Here's to working smarter and finding your flow.

Chapter 7

Habits and Routines – Your Daily Blueprint for Resilience

We've explored many tools and strategies for calming the nervous system and boosting resilience – now comes the challenge of weaving them seamlessly into your busy life. The answer lies in habits and routines. High-achieving people often rely on structured daily routines not because they're rigid or boring, but because routines reduce decision fatigue and ensure that the important things (like exercise, planning, family time) don't get pushed out by the merely urgent. By automating healthy behaviors, you free up mental energy and create a stable foundation for peak performance. In this chapter, we'll draw on well-known figures and behavioral science to help you design a daily blueprint that keeps you performing at your best *consistently*.

Consistent routines act like the scaffolding of a resilient life – they keep you steady even when work or life gets chaotic. It's easier to handle surprises and stress when your core habits (sleep, exercise, mindfulness, etc.) run on autopilot. Many successful leaders are *fanatical* about their daily schedules for exactly this reason. It's not about being inflexible; it's about proactively making space for what matters. As productivity expert James Clear puts it, "You do not rise to the level of your goals, you fall to the level of your systems." In other words, our habits determine our success. Let's look at how to build those habits into morning, workday, and evening routines that reinforce your resilience.

Morning Routines – Win the Morning, Win the Day

There's a popular saying: *win the morning, win the day*. Mornings are precious – a chance to set your mood, energy, and focus before the day's chaos hits. Many successful entrepreneurs and leaders have morning rituals to start the day on the right foot. For instance, peak-performance coach Tony Robbins famously begins his mornings with a priming routine that includes intense breathing exercises and a plunge into cold water. He might spend just a minute under a cold shower or in a cryotherapy pool, but that's enough to energize his physiology – the cold shock spikes his circulation and adrenaline, instantly waking him up. Robbins combines this with a short meditation and gratitude practice he calls "priming," which blends breathing techniques, visualization, and thanksgiving. In his words, this routine puts him in a *peak mental and emotional state* for the day ahead.

Others, like Apple's CEO Tim Cook, take a different approach – Cook is known to hit the gym as early as 5 a.m. to get the blood flowing. He wakes up well before dawn (around 4:00–4:30am) precisely because, as he says, the early morning is the part of the day he can "control the most" before emergencies arise. By 5:00 a.m., Cook is often doing an hour of strength training with a trainer. "I do no work during that period... I never check my phone, I'm just totally focused on working out," he notes – the workout not only keeps him fit but "helps keep my stress at bay". In short, exercise is non-negotiable in his morning routine.

Many other leaders carve out similar morning self-care: some practice meditation (for example, media mogul Oprah Winfrey centers herself with morning meditation), while others spend time reading or journaling before the day's meetings begin. The specifics can vary, but the common thread is carving out a proactive slice of time each morning devoted to self-care and intentional mindset, *before* you dive into emails, news, and other people's demands.

A neuroscience-backed addition to any morning routine is sunlight viewing. We touched on this in earlier chapters: getting outside in natural light shortly after waking has powerful effects on your biology. Exposure to morning sunlight (even just 5–10 minutes) triggers a cascade of hormonal signals that reset your circadian clock for the day. Sunlight hitting your eyes suppresses lingering melatonin (the sleep hormone) and triggers a healthy rise in cortisol, which actually helps you feel alert and awake. This cortisol spike, far from being "stressful," is a normal pulse known as the cortisol awakening response – it actually *lowers* stress later in the day by aligning your body clock. Morning sunlight also boosts serotonin, the neurotransmitter that improves mood (and later converts into melatonin at night to promote sleep). In fact, people who start getting morning light often report feeling noticeably more awake, happier, and then sleeping better that night. So, an easy win: step outside with your coffee or take a 10-minute stroll around the block each morning. You might combine habits here: for example, go for a short walk or light jog outdoors – this gives you movement (exercise), sunlight, and even a bit of mindfulness (enjoying some quiet or listening to birds) all at once. The key is *daylight* – indoor lighting is usually too dim to have the full effect, whereas real sunlight, even on a cloudy day, is potent. Think of morning light as nature's free energizer.

Another powerful morning habit is journaling or setting daily intentions. Many high-performers take a few minutes to write down 1–3 top priorities for the day, or to note a few things they're grateful for. Writing down priorities can give you clarity and focus – instead of immediately reacting to the world, you've declared what *you* intend to accomplish. Gratitude journaling, meanwhile, has been shown in positive psychology research to tangibly improve mood and even physical health. In studies, people who wrote down things they were grateful for each day saw boosts in emotional well-being, better sleep quality, and even improved biomarkers of health. As one Harvard report noted, gratitude practice is linked to *greater* emotional and social well-being, *better sleep* and *lower depression* – even a 9% reduction in risk of heart disease was observed in one long-term study of gratitude and health. Simply put, starting your morning by focusing on what's good in your life can set a positive tone that carries through stress later. Some people combine gratitude with goal-setting in a single journal entry – for example, writing "Today, I'm grateful for X, Y, Z, and my top priority is W." Even five minutes spent journaling in the morning can sharpen your mind and lift your spirits.

To summarize a "resilient" morning: proactivity is key. Rather than immediately scrolling on your phone or diving into a frenzy of emails, carve out a morning ritual that centers you. It could be: wake up, drink a glass of water, do 10 minutes of stretching or yoga, get outside for a brief walk in the sun, then shower and have a healthy breakfast. Or it could be:

make your bed, meditate for 5 minutes, take a cold shower, then journal with your coffee. There is no one "magic" routine for everyone – the magic is in *having* a routine that primes your body and mind for the day. By "winning the morning," you create momentum and reserve of calm that helps you handle whatever comes later.

Workday Routines – Manage Energy, Not Just Time

Once the workday begins, maintaining resilience becomes about managing your *energy* and focus, not just your time. Think of yourself as a sprinter, not a marathoner. Human energy naturally runs in cycles – we can only focus intensely for so long before our performance starts to decline. Rather than forcing yourself to power straight through hours on end (which often leads to diminishing returns and mistakes), it's far more effective to work in focused sprints of 60–90 minutes followed by a short break to recover. This pattern aligns with our ultradian rhythms (natural cycles of alertness) and has been validated by research. For example, a University of Illinois study found that even brief mental breaks can dramatically *improve* focus during a prolonged task. In that study, people who took two very short breaks during a 50-minute task maintained their performance to the end, whereas those who never took breaks saw their performance steadily decline. The brain benefits from switching gears momentarily – it's like hitting a reset button on your attention. After a 5-minute pause, you come back sharper.

You can build this rhythm of focus-and-break into a habit. One popular method is the Pomodoro technique (working ~25 minutes, then a 5-minute break, repeated). Or you might simply set a timer to remind you to stand, stretch, and take a few deep breaths every hour. Over time, this can become second nature – your body will start to *crave* those micro-breaks because it learns that a little movement or a yawn and stretch prevents the 3 p.m. burnout. The key is making breaks a regular part of your workflow, not something you only do when utterly exhausted. Treat breaks as investments in sustained productivity. During the break, you might step away from your screen, look out a window (resting your eyes), do a few shoulder rolls, or practice a minute of breathing exercises. Even a 5-minute walk to refill your water bottle can help. These pauses are not "lost time"; they're what keep your energy high and mind clear, so your next sprint of work is as good as the first.

Another powerful work habit is the "shutdown ritual" at day's end. In an always-connected world, many of us carry work stress into the evening – answering emails at the dinner table, lying in bed ruminating over projects. This prevents true recovery. Computer scientist and author Cal Newport suggests creating a strict routine to mentally close the work loop each day. For example, you might decide that at 6:00 p.m., you will spend your last 10 minutes organizing your to-do list for tomorrow, tidying your desk, and then say a phrase like "Shutdown complete" as you turn off your computer. Newport literally does this – he reviews his task list and calendar to ensure nothing critical is forgotten, then shuts his laptop and says "Schedule shutdown, complete". It's a cue to his brain that work is done. After that, if an intrusive work thought pops up, he reminds himself that he did his shutdown and everything is captured, so there's no need to dwell on it. This simple ritual led Newport to eliminate work-related stress in his evenings – he found he could truly relax once he trained his mind to trust the shutdown system. You can adopt your own version: perhaps a closing mantra, or a symbolic action like locking your office door, or writing the last email and saying "done for today." Some people change clothes when they finish work (swapping office attire for casual) as a physical signal of switching to personal time. The specific action isn't important – what's important is that you have a defined end to your workday routine. This helps you mentally disconnect so you can recharge.

During the workday, also consider habits that protect your focus. One example is scheduling meeting-free blocks for your most important work. If you have control over your calendar, you might block 9–11 a.m. (when many people's energy and creativity are highest) as a deep work zone – no meetings or calls, just focused work on your top priority task. Communicate this to colleagues if needed. Another habit is to batch process things like email at set times instead of constantly checking all day. For instance, you can decide to check email at 11:00 a.m. and 4:00 p.m., rather than letting it interrupt you continuously. This reduces distraction and decision-switching fatigue. Likewise, turning off non-essential notifications (or using "Do Not Disturb" mode) during focus periods can greatly enhance your productivity. By structuring your day into chunks – focus, then break; creative work, then reactive tasks – you are managing not just time but your mental energy.

Finally, remember to actually take a lunch break. It's easy to work through lunch, but even 20-30 minutes away from your desk to eat mindfully can rejuvenate you for the afternoon. If possible, avoid eating while working – you'll enjoy your food more and give your brain a true rest. A short walk after lunch or some sunlight can also fend off the post-lunch slump. These little routines (an afternoon walk, a 5 p.m. tidy-up, etc.) may seem minor, but they add up to a sustainable, resilient work rhythm. Instead of riding a rollercoaster of frantic activity and crashes, you establish a steady cadence of effort and recovery.

Evening Routines – Unplug and Recharge

The flip side of a productive morning is a calming evening. To sustain high performance, you need quality sleep and true down-time at night – which means an evening routine that helps you *unwind*. As we detailed in the sleep chapter, having a consistent wind-down ritual in the last 30–60 minutes before bed can dramatically improve your sleep quality. Think of it as landing a plane – you can't go from 100 mph to zero instantly; you have to gradually descend. Start by dimming the lights and shutting off stimulating screens. Bright light (especially blue light from phones/TVs) in the late evening tricks your brain into thinking it's daytime, suppressing melatonin. So, an hour before bed, consider the day done: work devices off, emails answered or left for tomorrow. Many families find it helpful to declare a "devices off by 9 PM" rule (adjust the time as needed) so that everyone gets into a quieter headspace.

What should you do in this wind-down period? Choose relaxing, low-stimulation activities that you enjoy. For some, this is reading fiction (nothing too intense or work-related). For others it could be gentle stretching, foam rolling tight muscles, or taking a warm shower. You might brew a cup of herbal tea. This is an excellent time for mindfulness practices that encourage deep relaxation. For example, you could do a 10-minute guided NSDR (Non-Sleep Deep Rest) protocol such as a yoga nidra meditation. Yoga nidra, often done lying down, systematically guides you through breathing and body awareness to induce a state of deep rest – almost like a power nap, but without falling fully asleep. Research shows that yoga nidra and similar NSDR practices can significantly reduce stress and anxiety, lower cortisol, and improve sleep quality. In one study, even in a corporate setting, a short daily yoga nidra session led to better sleep and psychological well-being for participants. Essentially, NSDR gives some of the restorative benefits of sleep in a short time, and it "trains" your nervous system to relax on demand. Doing this at bedtime can quiet a racing mind and prep you for a smoother transition into actual sleep.

If meditation isn't your thing, even practicing breath exercises can work wonders at night. Techniques like 4-7-8 breathing (inhale 4 seconds, hold 7, exhale 8) or simple belly breathing stimulate your vagus nerve and shift you into the parasympathetic "rest and digest" state. Gentle yoga or stretching can also release physical tension. Some people journal at night to offload worries – writing a few lines about your day or listing things you're grateful for can give a sense of closure. Choose whatever relaxes *you*. The important part is consistency: by doing the same sorts of relaxing cues each evening, you train your body and brain that *sleep is coming*. Over time, your system will start to wind down more easily because it recognizes "oh, it's after dinner and we're taking a slow walk, this means we're transitioning toward bed."

Speaking of which, if you have family, consider creating calming evening routines together. For example, an after-dinner family walk can serve multiple purposes: you get a little light cardio to aid digestion, you bond with loved ones (social connection reduces stress), and you gently lower the day's adrenaline. When you return, maybe everyone switches to quiet activities – reading, listening to soothing music, or chatting. Having a household "quiet hour" can help kids and adults alike prepare for sleep. And of course, try to keep the bedroom a sanctuary: dim, cool, and device-free. Scrolling social media or checking work email in bed is a quick recipe for a racing mind at midnight. Instead, maybe you listen to a short sleep story or do progressive muscle relaxation lying in bed.

By prioritizing these wind-down habits, you're protecting your sleep, which is arguably the most critical pillar of resilience. Sleep is when your body repairs itself and your brain clears waste and consolidates memories. As mentioned earlier, even top CEOs and athletes have learned to respect sleep as a performance enhancer – Amazon's Jeff Bezos famously insists on 8 hours of sleep, noting that if he shortchanges his sleep, he might get more hours to work but the quality of his decisions suffers. He believes good sleep is so vital that it's actually part of his duty to shareholders to be well-rested! In our culture, lack of sleep used to be worn as a badge of honor ("I'll sleep when I'm dead," "I only got 4 hours last night, look how hard I'm working"). Now, enlightened leaders realize that's nonsense – as LinkedIn's chief HR officer put it, bragging about getting by on 4–5 hours is basically admitting you're operating below par and harming your health. Science backs this up: cognitive performance peaks at around 7–8 hours of sleep for most adults, and declines if you go much below (or above) that. Chronic short sleep impairs attention, working memory, and decision-making. So, think of your evening routine as the guardian of your sleep – and by extension, the guardian of tomorrow's performance.

Habits 101 – Leveraging Behavioral Science

How do you actually build these new habits – morning exercise, hourly breaks, journaling, etc. – so that they stick? It's one thing to do something for a few days when motivation is high, but real change comes when the behavior becomes automatic. Here we turn to the science of habit formation. A helpful formula to remember is the ABCs: Anchor, Behavior, Reward. This comes from the work of Stanford behavior scientist BJ Fogg (and is echoed by James Clear in *Atomic Habits*). Here's how it works:

- **Anchor:** Choose an existing habit or obvious cue that will trigger the new behavior. The anchor can be a time of day ("after I wake up") or an event ("after I brush my teeth" or "when my 2:30pm alarm goes off"). It should be something you reliably do every day, so it serves as a solid reminder. For example, let "after I brew my morning coffee" be an anchor to do a 2-minute meditation. Or "when I return from lunch" be the anchor to do a quick stretch. Anchoring a new habit onto an old, established one is sometimes called habit stacking, a term popularized by James Clear. By piggybacking on an existing routine, you leverage the fact that your brain already has that sequence on autopilot. If you always make coffee at 7am, attaching "journal three things I'm grateful for" right after pouring the coffee makes it much more likely to happen (because the coffee routine will cue it).

- **Behavior:** This is the new habit itself – and when starting out, smaller is better. Design the behavior to be as easy and specific as possible, so there's minimal friction in doing it. For instance, instead of saying "I'll exercise every morning," the initial behavior could be "I will do 5 minutes of gentle yoga after brushing my teeth." Instead of "meditate daily," start with "after I sit at my desk, I'll take 3 deep breaths" or "I'll meditate for 2 minutes." Tiny behaviors might seem almost too trivial, but that's the point – if it's too easy to fail, you *won't* fail. You can always expand it later. Clear calls this the "two-minute rule" – any new habit should take under 2 minutes at first. On days when motivation is low or schedules crazy, you can still manage 2 minutes. That keeps the habit alive. Over weeks, you can scale up (2 minutes becomes 5, then 10, etc., or one set of exercise becomes two sets, and so on). Make sure the behavior is also specific: "exercise more" is vague; "do 20 squats at 5pm when my reminder chimes" is clear. Our brains like clear instructions.

- **Reward:** In the early stages of habit formation, it's important to give yourself a small reward or positive reinforcement immediately after the behavior. This helps your brain associate the habit with something good, activating the dopamine "habit loop." The reward doesn't have to be big – it could literally be saying "good job!" to yourself or checking off a habit tracker (which gives a little hit of satisfaction). Some people use other rewards like enjoying a cup of tea right after finishing their meditation, or playing a favorite song as they start their work break. Even the intrinsic good feeling from the behavior can be noted ("ah, that stretch felt nice!"). The key is to celebrate the win, no matter how small. Over time, the habit itself becomes rewarding because you'll feel the benefits (you start *craving* that relaxed feeling after meditation, or the endorphin rush after exercise). But in the beginning, consciously high-fiving yourself matters. As James Clear writes, each time you complete a habit, you are casting a vote for the identity you want – e.g. "I am a person who takes care of my mental fitness." Celebrating reinforces that identity.

Using these principles, you can *engineer* new routines step by step. Clear also advocates "habit stacking" as mentioned – essentially, the Anchor-Behavior technique above. For example: *After* I take off my work shoes in the evening (existing habit), I will *immediately* change into workout clothes (new habit). Or *after* I sit down with my morning coffee, I will *write my to-do list*. The beauty of habit stacking is that your current habits act as hooks – you don't have to remember a whole new schedule, you just insert the new action into an existing framework. And because the cue is tied to something solid (like coffee or toothbrushing), it's much easier to stay consistent. In one example, someone created a morning stack: 1) "After I pour my morning coffee, I will meditate for 60 seconds," 2) "After I meditate, I will write my top 3 priorities for the day," 3) "After I write my priorities, I will immediately start on the first one". This chain propels you right into a focused work session. The first link (coffee→meditate) is key – once that triggers, the rest can flow.

One more technique from Clear's *Atomic Habits* is focusing on identity over goals. Rather than saying "I want to run a 5K" (outcome-based), say "I'm becoming the kind of person who doesn't miss workouts." When a behavior ties into your sense of self, it sticks harder. Every time you do the habit, you reinforce an internal story: "I'm a meditator," "I'm a great sleeper," "I'm a family-first person who always has dinner with my kids." This mindset can supercharge habit formation because ultimately we act in alignment with who we believe we are. So embrace that identity *now* – even if you only meditate 2 minutes today, you can say, "I'm the type of person who meditates daily." It's not fake it till you make it; it's practice it until you become it.

Example – Designing John's Resilient Daily Routine

Let's illustrate how all these pieces can come together by imagining a composite character, John, a 45-year-old startup CTO who's been showing signs of burnout. John has been running on fumes: sleep-deprived, constantly anxious, scattered in his focus. He realizes he needs to course-correct and build more resilience through better habits. Here's how John redesigned his daily routine, step by step, to create a blueprint for stress-proof performance:

- **Morning (7:00–8:00 am):** John starts by waking at a consistent time. Upon waking, he makes his bed (a quick task that gives a small sense of accomplishment). Right *after* that, he spends 5 minutes journaling. He writes down his top 3 priorities for the day and a couple of things he's grateful for, anchoring this habit to after bed-making. This practice helps John cultivate a positive mindset and clarity on what matters most. Next, he does a 15-minute bodyweight workout on his patio – some push-ups, squats, and planks – which gets his blood flowing and, bonus, exposes him to morning sunlight. The natural light and exercise together energize him far more than the extra 15 minutes of hitting snooze used to. After a quick shower, John sits for 10 minutes of breathing exercises and meditation. He uses a guided app to keep it simple. By the time 8:00 rolls around, John has invested in his body (exercise), his mind (meditation), and his mood (gratitude journal) *before* the workday begins. He then has a high-protein breakfast (skipping the sugary pastry he used to grab, to avoid a mid-morning crash) and walks his kids to the bus stop. That short walk and chat with his kids doubles as family bonding and extra steps for his health. John arrives at work feeling focused and upbeat, instead of frazzled.

- **Workday (9:00 am–5:30 pm):** At work, John now structures his day intentionally. He communicated to his team that 9–11 am is a meeting-free focus block for him (barring true emergencies). During that time, he silences Slack and email notifications and dives into his most cognitively demanding work (for him, coding and strategic planning). He finds he gets more done in those two uninterrupted hours than he used to in half a day of stop-and-go work. Each hour, however, he practices the habit of taking a brief break – roughly at 10:00 and again at 11:00, he stands up to stretch and breathe for a few minutes. John set a Pomodoro timer on his computer that reminds him to "Stand up!" as the cue. This keeps his mind fresh (as that Illinois study suggested, the mini-breaks prevent decline in focus). By 11:00, he's accomplished deep work. He then spends 30 minutes (11–11:30) processing emails and Slack messages – batching them so it doesn't consume the whole day. Throughout the day, whenever John finishes a task or meeting, he quickly notes it down or updates his to-do list, staying organized. He also makes a point to take a real lunch break around 1:00 pm. Whereas before he'd munch a sandwich at his desk, now he steps away from his workspace to eat mindfully (sometimes joining a colleague or enjoying a book). Often, he'll take a 10-minute walk outside after lunch to get some sun and combat the post-lunch lull. The result is that his afternoon energy is much steadier. By 5:30 pm, an alarm on his phone goes off: this is John's cue to start closing out the workday. He'll review what tasks got done and quickly jot down any carryover tasks or notes for tomorrow (this clears his head so he won't worry about them later). He then performs his shutdown ritual: he closes his work apps, tidies his desk, and says "Done for the day" quietly to himself as he turns off the computer. This phrase, simple as it is, gives him a mental full-stop. Work is officially over. John leaves the office (or, on home-office days, shuts the office door) and shifts to personal time without the baggage of unresolved work angst.

- **Evening (after 6:00 pm):** In the evening, John has dinner with his family around 7:00 pm. He consciously avoids bringing his phone to the table or the bedroom, to minimize the temptation of late-night emails. After dinner, as a family they often take a short walk in the neighborhood if weather permits – this has become a cherished routine for connecting and unwinding. By 9:00 or 9:30 pm, John begins his wind-down routine. He dims the household lights and shuts off the TV and other bright screens. If he watches something with his spouse, it's a lighthearted show (no intense thrillers that spike adrenaline at 10 pm). Around 9:30, John might do 10 minutes of gentle yoga stretches or use a foam roller to release tension – this also helps with some back pain he's been addressing. If his mind is racing (perhaps thinking about an upcoming presentation), he'll lie in bed and play a 10-minute guided NSDR/yoga nidra audio which methodically relaxes his body and mind. By 10:00–10:15 pm, John is usually in bed and ready for sleep, aiming for roughly 7 hours of rest. He's set his environment for success: cool room, blackout curtains, no buzzing devices. Over the next few weeks, John notices he's falling asleep faster and waking up more refreshed, thanks to the consistency. His smartwatch data even shows his heart rate variability (HRV) trending upward, a sign of improved recovery. In the mornings, he no longer needs to drag himself out of bed after multiple snoozes – he often wakes up before the alarm, feeling *rested*.

John's routine might sound idealized – and indeed, life will inevitably throw curveballs. There will be days when a late emergency meeting cuts into his 5:30 shutdown, or nights when a sick child interrupts sleep. But because he's established these healthy pillars as his default, when disruptions happen he can rebound faster. If he has a bad night, he'll still do a gentle version of his morning routine, knowing it will help him recover. If work runs late one day, he'll still try to do a mini wind-down (maybe just 5 minutes of breathing) to signal his brain to sleep. In other words, the structure acts as a safety net. It keeps him from spiraling back into the old habits of working until 10pm, skipping workouts, and neglecting sleep. By sticking to his routine ~80% of the time, John finds that the occasional 20% chaos doesn't knock him off course anymore. He's more resilient to surprises because the healthy routine is his baseline. Over a few months, John's colleagues notice a change – he seems more calm and focused, even under pressure. John himself notices he's not reaching for a third cup of coffee in the afternoon and that the Sunday-night dread has reduced. This is the power of ingrained habits: they carry you through the rough days.

The Power of Incremental Change

A final note: you don't need to overhaul your entire life overnight. In fact, please don't try to. The surest path to failure is taking on too much change at once ("Tomorrow I will start a 5am workout, 30-minute meditation, completely new diet, 4 major work habits... and never watch TV again"). That's a recipe for overwhelm. Instead, embrace the power of small, incremental improvements – the "1% better" philosophy.

Choose one habit from this chapter that resonated with you – something that feels most feasible or impactful for your situation. Maybe it's "shut down work by 6pm and be present with family," or "do 10 minutes of mindfulness each morning," or "walk for 15 minutes every afternoon." Implement it consistently for a few weeks. Once it starts to feel natural (or at least less of a struggle), layer on another habit. These modest 1% upgrades may seem insignificant day to day, but they compound over time. As author James Clear points out, tiny gains sustained over a long period can lead to remarkable results. To use his math: getting just 1% better each day for a year doesn't make you 365% better – due to compounding, it actually makes you about 37 times better by year's end (in whatever metric you're measuring). Now, in real life, personal growth isn't so easily quantifiable, but the core idea holds: small changes, repeated consistently, lead to massive improvement down the line.

Even if you're improving at, say, 1% per week, in a year that's roughly a 67% improvement – which is huge! Imagine being even 30% better at managing stress and sustaining your performance a year from now – you'd notice the difference. We have real-world evidence of these kinds of gains. For example, when the insurance company Aetna offered a mindfulness program to employees, those who participated saw stress levels drop by 28% on average and gained about 62 minutes of productivity per week. That's a concrete illustration that dedicating time to wellness habits can make you substantially more effective. Another example: a study of executives who improved their sleep hygiene found corresponding boosts in productivity and decision-making accuracy (sleep really is a secret weapon for productivity). The point is, these *incremental changes* in daily routine create a positive feedback loop. As you feel better and more in control, you're motivated to continue, and you might add another habit. Over months, you may find you've transformed your routine and your resilience in ways that would have overwhelmed you if attempted all at once.

So, start small. Pick one thing and do it this week. Celebrate that. Next week or next month, pick another. Patience is key – you're trying to create *sustainable habits*, not quick fixes. And don't beat yourself up for slip-ups. Missing one day is fine; just get back on track the next day (what Clear calls never missing twice). Those small wins will accumulate. In a year, you might look back and be astonished at how far you've come – perhaps you're sleeping better, your mood is brighter, your focus at work sharper, your body stronger. And importantly, you'll likely feel more in control and fulfilled, not just more "efficient." After all, the goal of all these habits is not to turn you into some productivity robot, but to help you thrive with less stress and more satisfaction.

Conclusion: Thriving Amid Stress – Your New Normal

Chronic stress and burnout are formidable challenges of our era, especially in high-performance careers. But they are *not* unbeatable. By applying the principles in this guide – listening to your body's signals, prioritizing sleep and recovery, practicing mindfulness, nurturing your physical health, and optimizing how you work – you can transform stress from a destructive force into a catalyst for growth. The goal isn't to live a life completely free of stress (that's neither possible nor desirable, since some stress in small doses keeps us sharp). Rather, the goal is to build so much resilience that you can navigate high-pressure situations with agility and poise. When a challenge arises, it doesn't knock you down for long – you have the habits and tools to respond, recover, and even learn from it.

Think of yourself as a corporate athlete. Just as elite athletes cycle through intensive training and deliberate recovery to maximize performance, you too can cycle through periods of focused work and periods of rest and renewal. No athlete in the world trains 12 hours a day, 7 days a week – they would collapse. Instead, they balance strain and recovery, because the recovery is when growth happens (muscles rebuild, skills consolidate). In the corporate world, many of us forgot that principle. We tried to be "always on," and we paid the price with chronic fatigue, burnout, and declining effectiveness. Now it's time to reclaim the athlete's mindset: treat your *mind and body* with the same care a pro athlete treats theirs. That means valuing sleep, nutrition, exercise, and mental focus as foundational pieces of your job. When you do, you'll actually gain a competitive edge in your professional arena. You'll make better decisions, be more creative, and have more endurance when it counts. And beyond the KPIs and achievements, you'll likely discover something even more rewarding – a better quality of life. When you're well-rested, mentally centered, and physically healthy, work doesn't consume you or diminish you. It becomes more enjoyable and sustainable. You show up not just as a better executive or entrepreneur, but as a better parent, partner, friend, and human being.

Let's recap a few key takeaways and action points as you move forward into your new normal:

- **Burnout is real – monitor your stress like a metric.** Don't ignore signs of chronic stress or wear it as a badge of honor. Acknowledge it and course-correct early. If you like data, use tools like heart rate variability trackers to get objective feedback – changes in HRV can be an early warning sign from your nervous system that you're overloaded. Even without gadgets, practice self-awareness: check in with yourself regularly (maybe during those breaks). If you notice persistent exhaustion or apathy, that's a signal to prioritize recovery, not just "push through." Remember, burnout is not a failure of character; it's often a mismatch between demands and rest. It's correctable once recognized.

- **Sleep is non-negotiable – protect your 7–8 hours like a meeting with your CEO.** Overwhelming evidence shows sleep is a superpower for performance. Think of it as your secret productivity weapon: good sleep literally improves memory, creativity, and cognitive speed. It also stabilizes your mood and energy (ever notice how problems feel 10x worse after a bad night's sleep?). Prioritize sleep by keeping consistent bed and wake times, creating a wind-down routine, and making your sleep environment comfortable. If you must choose, it's better to sacrifice an hour of late-night work for an hour of sleep – you'll likely make up that productivity (and then some) the next day with a clearer brain. As Jeff Bezos quipped, "If you shortchange your sleep, you might get a couple of extra 'productive' hours, but that productivity might be an illusion". Quality over quantity. Treat sleep as sacred.

- **Mindfulness and breaks are productivity enhancers, not hindrances.** Train your brain with practices like meditation, and give it brief breaks to recharge focus. Even just 5–10 minutes of meditation or breathing a day can rewire your stress response and improve concentration – studies have shown that as little as 20 minutes a day for two months leads to measurably better focus and less anxiety. And remember the power of stepping away: doing something as simple as a 5-minute break each hour or a short walk in the afternoon can prevent mental fatigue and keep your work quality high. Don't feel guilty for taking breaks – realize that rest is part of work. A rested brain is a more effective brain. In the long run, you get more done, not less.

- **Exercise and diet matter for your mind as much as your body.** We often compartmentalize physical health from mental health, but they are deeply connected. Regular movement boosts your brain chemistry in profoundly positive ways. Exercise releases endorphins (natural mood lifters) and increases levels of BDNF, a neurotrophic factor often called "Miracle-Gro for the brain" that promotes neuron growth and connectivity. In one vivid analogy, BDNF is like fertilizer that helps your brain sprout new cells and neural pathways, which improves learning and memory. This is partly why exercise is linked to better mood and

121

lower rates of depression. You don't need to become a triathlete – even a brisk 20-minute walk or a bike ride a few times a week can confer benefits. The key is consistency. Likewise, how you fuel yourself impacts your mental state. Eat in a way that supports stable energy and focus: for example, heavy processed carbs at lunch might lead to a crash, whereas a balance of protein, healthy fats, and complex carbs will sustain you. Staying hydrated and limiting excessive caffeine or alcohol (which can mess with sleep and mood) also goes a long way. Essentially, treat your body like the vehicle for your ambitions – premium fuel, regular maintenance, and it will carry you further.

- **Work smarter, not just harder.** It's a cliché, but in the context of resilience it means embracing strategies like single-tasking (give full attention to one thing at a time), finding your flow state (that zone of intensive focus which is deeply satisfying), and not being afraid to unplug to recover. Your best work often comes after a period of rejuvenation. Think about when you get your best ideas – maybe on a walk, or in the shower, or during a weekend off. Constant grind actually diminishes creativity and strategic thinking. So, set boundaries to protect deep work and personal time. Use those boundaries not as limitations but as productivity hacks – when you're working, you're *fully on*, and when you're resting, you're *fully off*. This oscillation ensures you bring your A-game when it counts. It also means learning to delegate, prioritize, or even say no when necessary, so you're directing your effort where it truly matters rather than spinning wheels on trivial tasks.

High performers often distinguish themselves not by doing *more* of everything, but by doing *more of the right things* and allowing recovery to sharpen their edge.

- **Routines build resilience.** This entire chapter has hammered this point: by establishing daily habits that automate self-care and recovery, you create a buffer against stress. When big challenges arrive, you're *grounded by routine*. It's like a well-trained martial artist who, in a fight, instinctively falls back on trained stances and breathing – rather than panic, they respond from muscle memory. Similarly, if you've ingrained habits like taking calming breaths when tense, or stepping away from conflict to cool down, those will kick in during crisis moments. Routines in sleep, exercise, planning, and relaxation ensure that the fundamentals of your well-being are always being maintained. This consistency is your secret weapon. It means on a tough day, you still ate a decent breakfast and took a walk, so you're better equipped to handle the stressor than if you'd skipped meals and sat hunched over a desk for 10 hours. Over time, the routine essentially raises your baseline – you operate at a higher default level of resilience and performance, so you're less rattled by spikes in stress.

Remember the story of Arianna Huffington, who we mentioned earlier. In 2007, she was burning the candle at both ends running the Huffington Post, until one day she literally collapsed from exhaustion – broke her cheekbone on the way down – a wake-up call that made her reassess her approach to success. She realized that achievement at the cost of health isn't true success at all. Arianna transformed her collapse into a crusade for a better way of working. She wrote books on wellbeing (*Thrive* and *The Sleep Revolution*) and founded Thrive Global, a company dedicated to ending the burnout culture. In her own words, "that day changed my life. It put me on a course where I changed how I work and how I live". Now she advocates for sleep, meditation, and balance in workplaces worldwide. Or consider the example of the Aetna employees we just discussed, who became more productive only after their CEO encouraged mindfulness and healthier work habits. When over 13,000 Aetna employees took part in yoga and meditation classes, they averaged a 28% stress reduction and gained an extra 62 minutes of productivity per week. These aren't fluffy, feel-good anecdotes – they're hard data showing that well-being fuels performance. As Arianna often says, it's not about simply surviving the grind, but *thriving* and actually getting better results. When you take care of your body and brain, they take care of your business and ambitions in return.

As you implement these strategies in your own life, be patient and kind to yourself. Behavior change is a journey, not a switch. There will be days you fall off the wagon – that's okay. What matters is getting back on more times than you fall off. Celebrate progress, not perfection. If you meditated 3 days this week instead of 0 last week, that's a win – don't focus on the 4 days you didn't. Each positive action is an investment in the new, resilient you. And perhaps you'll inspire those around you as well. We're seeing a shift in many high-performance cultures: from the old 24/7 hustle ethos toward a more enlightened model that values wellness as the foundation of excellence. By living this example, you become a role model for a healthier definition of success. It might start with you encouraging your team to take lunch breaks, or sharing how prioritizing sleep actually helped you finish a project faster. These small cultural changes can ripple outward.

In the end, the aim is not just to survive the demands of modern professional life, but to thrive – to achieve sustained high performance *while also* enjoying the ride. Life's too short and careers too long to burn out early. Stress will always be part of the picture in some form; the world moves fast and challenges will come. But now you have the tools to meet it head-on: to harness the useful energy of stress when needed, and to mitigate its harms when it's not. You've learned to reset your nervous system, to cultivate habits that make you stronger and more centered. This is your new normal – one where peak performance and well-being coexist.

Here's to your journey from burnout to peak performance. May you achieve success *with* satisfaction and strength, not at the cost of them. With your daily resilience blueprint in hand, you're ready to thrive amid stress, not in spite of it. Go forth and make your new normal a reality – one habit, one day at a time. You've got this.

Epilogue

You now hold the keys to your most powerful ally: your vagus nerve. Through these pages, you've discovered how this remarkable tenth cranial nerve serves as the master conductor of your autonomic orchestra, orchestrating everything from your heart rate variability to your capacity for deep, restorative calm.

The science has shown you that peak performance stems not from pushing harder, but from cultivating the subtle art of nervous system regulation. Every breathing technique you've learned, every cold exposure protocol you've practiced, and every mindfulness exercise you've integrated has been quietly rewiring your neural pathways, strengthening your vagal tone like building muscle fiber by fiber.

Your stress response system no longer controls you—you control it. The chronic fight-or-flight patterns that once drained your energy and clouded your focus have given way to a more flexible, resilient nervous system. You can now access states of calm alertness that seemed impossible before, maintaining clarity under pressure while preserving your vitality for what matters most.

The transformation extends far beyond individual techniques. You've learned to read your body's signals with newfound precision, recognizing the early whispers of stress before they become overwhelming storms.

This awareness has become your compass, guiding you toward choices that support rather than sabotage your well-being.

Your nervous system reset journey continues with every conscious breath, every moment of presence, every choice to respond rather than react. The tools are yours now—tried, tested, and backed by decades of neuroscientific research. Your vagus nerve stands ready to support your highest aspirations, your deepest creativity, and your most meaningful work.

The future belongs to those who understand that true strength flows from inner harmony. That future is yours.

www.ingramcontent.com/pod-product-compliance
Lightning Source LLC
Chambersburg PA
CBHW070121030426
42335CB00016B/2229